Bach Flower Remedies for your horse

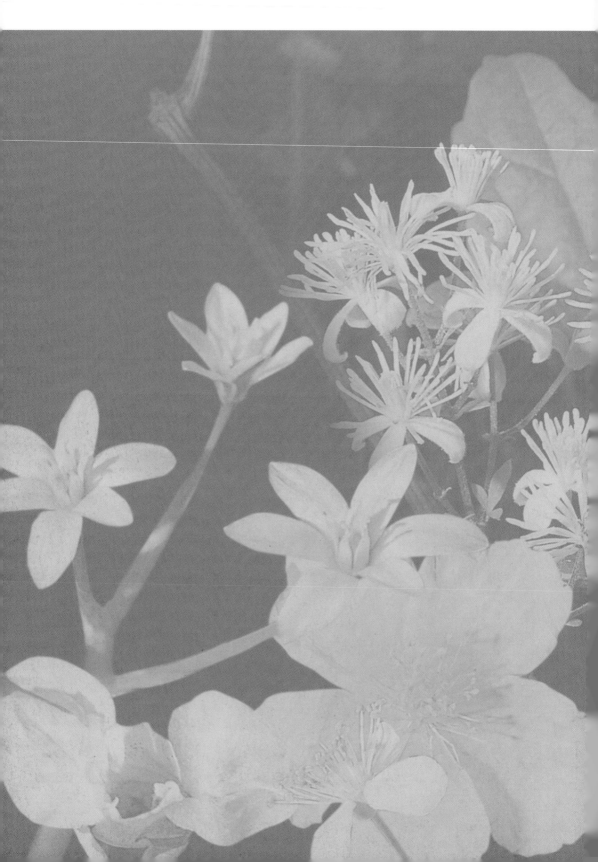

Bach Flower
Remedies
for your horse

Reducing stress and alleviating symptoms

By Marion Brehmer

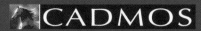

Copyright of german edition: © 2005 by Cadmos Verlag
Copyright of this edition: © 2006 by Cadmos Equestrian
Arrangement and setting: Ravenstein and Partners, Verden
Cover photograph: Christiane Slawik
Printing: Westermann, Zwickau

Printed in Germany

ISBN 3-86127-921-5

Contents

A-Z of problems suggested treatments

Proven Bach Flower remedies and mixtures for common problems

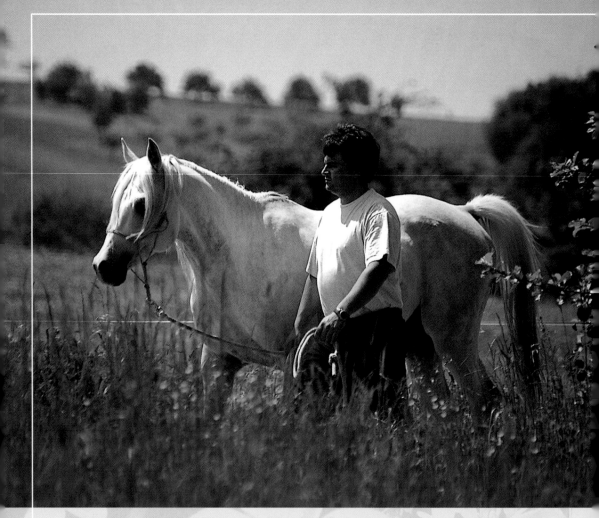

Harmony between man and horse can only exist if we are aware of the horse's fundamental needs and take these into account in all dealings with the animal. Photo: Schmelzer

Introduction

Man and horse have shared an incomparably close relationship that has spanned thousands of years. This relationship has grown over the course of the history of civilisation and is often very emotionally charged in our present day. However, the horse, that has become man's companion in both sport-

ing and leisure activities, is intrinsically a herd animal, instinctively poised for flight and man still needs to manage the horse in a way that caters for all his needs. Many riding establishments are opposed to recent developments in horse management that advocate the use of open stables and the practice of regularly turning horses out into the field. Several of them continue to allow their horses to spend most of their day in stables, which are only a few metres wide. Keeping a horse in these conditions, in which the only diversion offered is the daily ride and feed, can lead to common allergies, behaviour disorders and bad habits. If the fundamental needs of the horse are not being met and the horse is inappropriately managed, psychological disturbances can develop. These are then expressed as anxiety, nervousness or aggression towards people and other horses, stereotypical behaviour like windsucking or weaving or an increased susceptibility to illnesses.

To resolve these problems successfully in the long term, it is essential to manage the horse in a way that corresponds to his natural instincts and fulfils all his needs. This should allow the owner to discover the true nature of the horse, without being unduly influenced by his own anthropomorphic views and it can help him to prevent abnormal behaviour patterns developing. In conjunction with this, using Bach Flower remedies can help to restore the overall balance of body and soul in a safe way, free from side effects.

Bach Flowers influence the spirit. They regulate negative vibrations and produce a harmonious balance. If a situation arises in which a horse needs to be calmed – for example, following a shock, a negative experience or because of deep-rooted psychological disturbances – giving the correct combination of Bach Flower remedies can be invaluable. Anxiety and aggression can be eliminated, self-confidence can be re-established and symptoms of shock involving feelings of grief or jealousy can be alleviated. Rescue Remedy – the so-called drops to be taken in an emergency (see page 75) – should be present in every stable first-aid kit for acute situations.

Bach Flowers can have a dramatic effect on the immune system by activating positive energy. They are not intended to be used instead of consulting a vet when the horse is ill but rather to balance out the disharmonies that can lead to an organic illness or which are triggered through an illness.

Bach Flowers remedies are eminently suitable for treating psychological imbalances. This book shows the variety of ways in which Bach Flower remedies can be used, together with detailed portraits of the 38 flowers. It also offers essential information on the fascinating plant essences obtained through well-researched data. The book provides fundamental knowledge for the interested horse owner that will enable him to select the right combination of Bach Flowers.

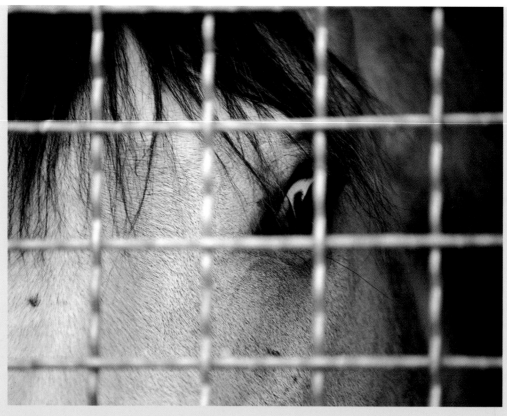

Bach Flowers help to restore the horse's psychological equilibrium - provided that his fundamental needs are being met i.e. that he is being correctly managed. Photo: Schmelzer

Bach Flower remedies are unable to solve psychological problems if there are significant shortcomings in the way the horse is managed. Every horse owner should provide the best possible living conditions for their horse. Daily contact with other horses as well as a balanced diet that takes into account all the needs of the horse are vital. In addition to this, psychological damage can occur if excessive demands are constantly placed on the horse in competitions and this can result in later physical illnesses.

Bach Flowers

The flowers and the way they work

Bach Flowers are essences that are produced from specially selected wild flowers, trees and bushes by natural means. Strictly speaking the number of 38 Bach Flowers comes from 37 flower essences and Rock Water essence. Their names are derived from the English Doctor Edward Bach, who discovered the effects of the essences between 1930 and 1936 and used them in treating patients suffering from distinct negative states of mind – for example from anxiety, aggression, despair and uncertainty. According to Bach these negative emotional disturbances are the reasons why the patients became ill in the first place. It is generally acknowledged that to some extent, extreme psychological pressure leaves the way wide open for illnesses. An illness often arises precisely when the patient is psychologically unstable as a result of negative influences. The immune system is weakened and the body does not seem to have enough strength to defend itself against the attack.

Once the state of mind becomes stable, the body's own ability to heal itself improves and the illness can be cured more easily and more rapidly. Bach Flower remedies are able to help the patient to return to a state of psychological balance and in the process eliminate the physical symptoms.

There also exists a very close connection between psychological imbalance and physical as well as psychological disturbances in animals. Practise has shown that animals often respond particularly swiftly to the positive impulses of Bach Flowers so that equilibrium can be restored within a very short space of time. Above all, excellent results can be obtained from using Bach Flower remedies in dealing with acute psychological disturbances and marked behavioural problems (anxiety, aggression, problems within the herd, training difficulties). They are effective in all types of emergencies and as a form of psychological support in difficult situations (visits from the farrier, transportation, birth, grief). They have also been successfully used to accompany the treatment of chronic conditions such as diarrhoea, eczema or allergies.

If a horse is showing signs of seemingly inexplicable behaviour, which is not linked to any physical disturbances, inspecting his immediate vicinity can often provide clues as to the cause of the problem. Horses relate to their environment in different ways and their behaviour often reflects conflict with other members of the herd or with the people who look after them. Their behaviour can be influenced in this way by several other factors including a change of stable, a new neighbour or building work carried out in the areas the horse visits.

What the owner of the animal experiences is possibly a psychological cry for help from the horse. Experienced animal therapists always try to obtain an exact picture of the animal's environment and lifestyle. At the same time as treating the horse, it is often useful to give a suitable Bach Flower remedy to the people who are dealing with the horse (such as the owner or rider).

In order to establish a harmonious relationship between man and animal it is often useful to treat not only the horse but also the people with whom the horse comes into contact by giving them both a suitable Bach Flower remedy. Selecting the appropriate Bach Flowers for humans can be done with the help of existing literature or by consulting a practitioner specialising in Bach Flowers remedies.

Bach Flowers can be used:

- In emergencies and in cases of acute psychological tension.
- For long-term chronic conditions and to combat impatience or irritability.
- As a remedy for psychological behaviour disorders.
- As support in training, during difficulties when being ridden and for any problems when in contact with the horse.

Dr. Edward Bach

"Disease is the means adopted by our own souls to point out to us our faults, to hinder us from doing more harm and to bring us back to the path of Truth and Light from which we never should have strayed"

Dr. Edward Bach

During his lifetime, Dr. Edward Bach (1886 – 1936) was a well-known doctor of immunology, bacteriology and pathology in England. While working as an assistant at the Bacteriological Institute at the University Clinic in London he came across seven groups of intestinal bacteria which, according to his observations, were connected to the onset of chronic diseases. These bacteria were also to be found in the intestines of healthy people. However in those with chronic diseases they were greatly increased. As a trial he isolated these bacteria from the stool of a sick patient and created vaccines from it, which he then injected into the same people, irrespective of the type of illness they were suffering from. The healing results achieved in this manner were astonishing. Not only did the general health of the patients improve as a result but there were also marked improvements in chronic conditions such as arthritis, rheumatism and headaches, or else the complaint disappeared altogether. However, these remedies sometimes caused painful reactions, so Bach swiftly set out to discover alternative means of using them. He later came in contact with the homeopath Samuel Hahnemann and thereafter began to increase the bacteria cultures according to homeopathic procedures. He prescribed the nosode preparations produced in this way to be taken internally. The outcome far surpassed the results achieved with the injections and made it much easier to actually take the remedies at the same time. This new method was the source of much interest in medical circles and was also prescribed in America, Germany and numerous other countries.

In addition to the clear physical effect of the homeopathic preparations that he had developed, Bach was also interested in discovering how the emotional symptoms accompanying the illness had altered. He established the fact that each of the seven groups of bacteria has an effect on a well-defined personality type. In this way, merely through observing the behaviour and symptoms exhibited by the patients, he was gradually able to draw conclusions as to the predominant groups of bacteria and prescribe the corresponding nosode preparations.

Despite the enormous success of this healing method, Bach was still not entirely satisfied with his work. For one thing he didn't want to work with the substances produced from the illness itself (the prepared intestinal bacteria) permanently and

was searching for an alternative from the plant world. For another thing, he perceived illness as the result of disharmony between the body and soul of man and he began to look into possibilities for treating the actual causes in the realm of feelings. In order to devote himself to his research, he eventually gave up his practice in London and moved to the country.

With his strongly defined sensitivity, within six years of being there he had discovered 37 plants, as well as an essence from water, with strong healing powers. Their vibrations corresponded to 38 archetypal human states of mind. Firstly he discovered the so-called 12 healers: Agrimony, Centaury, Cerato, Chicory, Clematis, Gentian, Impatiens, Mimulus, Scleranthus, Rock Rose, Vervain and Water Violet. Bach consequently found that these 12 flowers alone did not always lead to a satisfactory outcome in persistent cases. Living beings that have accepted their fate required stronger plants – plants that dominate the land-scape in large quantities or tall, richly coloured ones. Bach found seven further essences to be the so-called seven helpers, essences that also featured strongly in customs and Celtic traditions: Gorse, Heather, Oak, Olive, Rock Water, Vine and Wild Oat. Bach gradually discovered the remaining 19 flowers that could react with essences of the same frequency to the varying states of mind.

Bach made use of simple potency procedures and fell back on the traditional methods, which the Indians had already used for their plants. The highly expensive potency procedures proved to be unsuitable for producing healing methods from the flowers.

The seven main groups

Dr. Bach arranged all problematic emotional states of mind into seven main groups with corresponding flowers for each one. To supplement the treatment of emotional problems different 'helper flowers' can be used that make up the correct mixture for the individual, according to the character and emotional condition.

---

1. Fear (Aspen, Cherry Plum, Mimulus, Red Chestnut, Rock Rose)

Negative emotional conditions and their positive transformation:
- Panic – Rock Rose takes care of presence of mind
- Fear of known things – Mimulus inspires courage
- Fear of mind giving way – Cherry Plum brings calmness
- Fears of unknown origin – Aspen deals with vague fear
- Fear or over concern for others – Red Chestnut promotes independence

---

2. Uncertainty (Cerato, Gentian, Gorse, Hornbeam, Scleranthus, Wild Oat)

Negative emotional conditions and their positive transformation:
- Weakness of judgement – Cerato promotes intuition
- Inner conflict – Scleranthus gives strength in making decisions
- Pessimism – Gentian strengthens confidence
- Despair – Gorse gives hope
- Mental lethargy – Hornbeam provides impetus
- Disorientation – Wild Oat brings determination

---

3. Insufficient interest in the present (Clematis, Chestnut Bud, Honeysuckle, Mustard, Olive, White Chestnut, Wild Rose)

Negative emotional conditions and their positive transformation:
- Mental escapism – Clematis restores a sense of reality
- Idealisation of the past – Honeysuckle promotes an awareness of the present
- Resignation – Wild Rose strengthens a zest for life
- Unwanted thoughts – White Chestnut provides inner balance
- Sadness, depression – Mustard gives "inner light"
- Failure to learn from mistakes in the past – Chestnut Bud promotes the ability to learn

4. Loneliness (Heather, Impatiens, Water Violet)

Negative emotional conditions and their positive transformation:

- Isolation – Water Violet promotes the ability to form relationships
- Impatience, hectic pace – Impatiens strengthens patience
- Self-centredness – Heather provides empathy

5. Over sensitivity (Agrimony, Centaury, Holly, Walnut)

Negative emotional conditions and their positive transformation:

- Obsession with harmony – Agrimony promotes the ability to deal with conflict
- Weakness of will – Centaury gives will-power
- Easily influenced by others – Walnut provides adaptability
- Jealousy, hatred – Holly opens the heart

6. Despondency and despair
(Crab Apple, Elm, Larch, Pine, Star of Bethlehem, Sweet Chestnut, Willow)

Negative emotional conditions and their positive transformation:

- Lack of self-confidence – Larch promotes feelings of self worth
- Self-reproach, guilt – Pine regulates self-respect
- Stress – Elm gives inner confidence
- Utter despair – Sweet Chestnut provides relief
- Trauma – Star of Bethlehem comforts the soul
- Resentment – Willow gives a sense of responsibility for the self
- False feelings of duty – Oak helps to provide a more appropriate sense of perseverance
- Susceptibility to infection – Crab Apple helps to promote order and cleanliness

7. Excessive care for the welfare of others (Beech, Chicory, Rock Water, Vervain, Vine)

Negative emotional conditions and their positive transformation:

- Selfishly possessive – Chicory offers love without condition
- Over-exuberance – Vervain promotes an ability to show enthusiasm
- Strong-willed – Vine provides authority within
- Obsessive criticism, intolerance – Beech strengthens tolerance
- Severity towards self, inner tension – Rock Water helps with flexibility

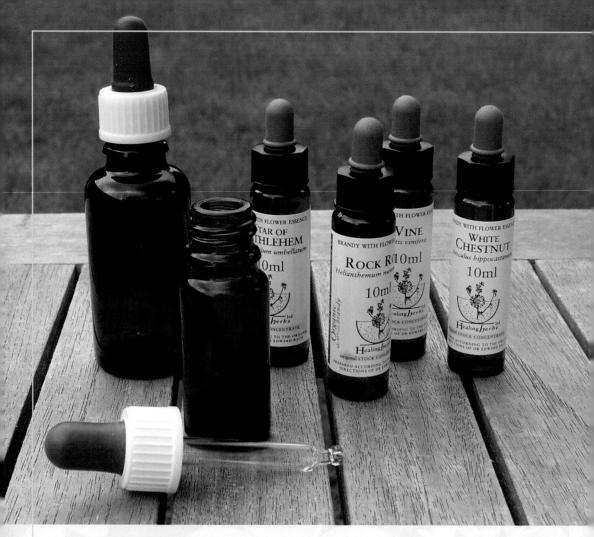

Use and dosage

Preparing a dispensing bottle

To prepare a Bach Flower mixture yourself you will need:

- The concentrates (the so-called stock bottles) of the selected flowers,

- A 20ml or 30 ml bottle with a pipette or dropper lid,
- Pure, still water.

You do not need to use alcohol or vinegar as an extra preservative when giving the mixtures to animals due to the fact that they will not take it.

Add one drop of the selected flower essence to 10ml of still water. If you are using a 30ml bottle add three drops of the concentrate per flower to the water. If only one flower is being used then add two drops for every 10ml of water.

Depending on the situation, several flowers can be freely mixed together. Experience has shown that that the "prescribed" limit of up to six flowers is not always useful. In certain cases a large number of flowers can be used perfectly well, sometimes just one or two flowers suffice.

The stock bottles should be stored at room temperature and, as far as possible, kept away from light and electrical appliances (computers, microwaves). The expiry date given is a mere formality. As the energetic qualities are maintained within, there should be no limit as to how long the stock bottles will last if stored appropriately.

Dosage

Bach Flowers work on energy not by means of prescribed methods. Higher doses do not have a greater effect than the quantities recommended in the box, right. Since Bach Flower remedies, as a homeopathic treatment, are absorbed most quickly through the mucous membrane of the mouth, please note the following points:
• If possible, do not give the animal the Bach Flower remedies with food or water but instead place directly in the mouth or on a piece of apple, carrot or dry bread.

• Give out the remedies before feeding times.
• If your horse is receiving any other treatment i.e. homeopathic medication, do not administer both items at the same time. Leave a gap of at least 15 minutes between the two.

If you have not been advised by your therapist as to the correct dosage of Bach Flowers, use the following as guidelines:
Foals and ponies 2-3 times daily 2-5 drops
Large horses 2 –3 times daily 5-8 drops
Rescue remedy can be given in slightly higher dosages (6-8 drops for foals and ponies and 8-10 drops for large horses) and in acute cases up to 4 times an hour until the situation has improved. As the symptoms fade do not suddenly stop administering the Bach Flower remedies altogether but gradually reduce the amount given. With a dosage of 5 drops twice daily, the ideal is to reduce it to 4 drops twice a day for the next two days and then for the following two days to reduce it to 3 drops and then 2 drops twice a day.

As with homeopathy, initially intense physical or psychological reactions to the remedies (referred to as the initial worsening) are a positive sign as they signal the energetic system's ability to respond and the beginning of the healing process. First reactions may include a need for more sleep, restlessness, diarrhoea or a lack of interest in normal activities.

These reactions normally disappear within one or two days. Since horses as individuals respond in different ways, there may well not be any initial reactions at all. Thus the absence of any discernible reaction does not indicate an error in your choice of flowers.

The alternative: Bach Flower remedies in the form of globules

There is an alternative to the essences based on alcohol solutions, created especially for use with animals, and this is in the form of small tablets made out of saccharine (globules). A company called Miraflowers now produces globules, which have been created according to Edward Bach's specifications concerning the watery extracts (original essences) of the relevant plants. The effectiveness of the MiraPet globules is in keeping with the classical Bach Flower essences. Their advantages lie in the absence of alcohol and the ease with which they can be given to animals. Simply place the globules in the corner of the mouth – the energetic information is then passed directly through the mucous membrane. Alternatively, the globules can be inserted into a piece of apple or something similar and administered in this way.

In terms of dosage for ponies and large horses, the manufacturer recommends six globules for each Bach Flower remedy, four times daily. From an organisational point of view, this can prove quite difficult to follow through for many horse owners. Experience has shown that giving the globules once a day and, if possible, a second dose in food or drinking water is perfectly satisfactory.

Length of therapy

In principle Bach Flower remedies should be given for as long as the horse is showing symptoms that require treatment. Bach Flower remedies often work very quickly, even though long-standing problems may require a bit of patience until the desired change in behaviour becomes apparent. How long you should persist in using a Bach Flower remedy varies in different cases. It is generally recommended that you continue for an initial period of two to four weeks from the first dose given. After that you should consult the therapist and, if necessary, change the remedy.

If no changes are evident within the first 14 days of taking the remedy, the choice of flowers should be reconsidered. The person observing the horse's behaviour does not always provide a totally objective report and it is often necessary to do a little bit of detective work in order to judge the psychological needs of the horse correctly.

In certain circumstances in dealing with long-term treatment it is sometimes necessary to change the emphasis if an underlying problem is gradually exposed. In these cases it is important to check to see if the composition of the Bach Flower remedy is still valid after a maximum of four weeks and to change it accordingly if necessary.

Generally speaking, three types of therapy have been established:
• Acute therapy: This is recommended for critical and sudden displays of disturbed behaviour or psychological problems, to be given for an initial period from one day to up to two weeks. Often only one or very few flowers are used
• Long-term therapy: In this case the emphasis is on treating disturbances that have already been in place for a long time. The Bach Flower remedies are

normally given over a period of several months or even a year. Several flowers are usually required. The combination of flowers should be reviewed after two to four weeks and altered according to any changes in the horse's mood.

• Permanent therapy: This course of action is chosen if the horse shows tendencies to revert to old behaviour patterns after taking the remedy.

Usage in conjunction with homeopathic treatments and medicines

Bach Flower remedies are free from side effects and will have no impact at all on any other forms of treatment. They can therefore be freely taken at the same time as other medication and, of course, homeopathic remedies. Leave a gap of at least 15 minutes between giving different forms of treatment.

Bach Flower remedies as a means of doping?

The regulations surrounding doping in equestrian sports events are currently extraordinarily strict. There is a long list of medication and active substances which if found to be present in a horse upon testing - even in very dilute quantities – can result in elimination from the competition and can lead to action being taken against the owner.

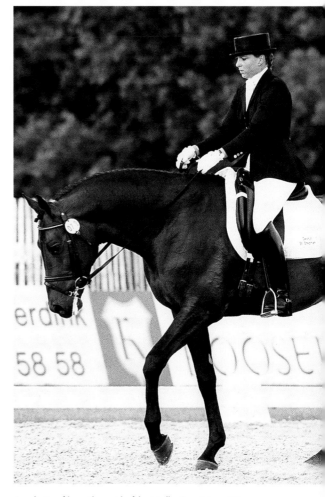

In order to safely avoid any risk of doping allegations at competitions you should stop giving the horse Bach Flower remedies in the form of alcoholic drops at least two days prior to the event and give them in globule form instead. Photo: Ernst

Bach Flower remedies do not have a chemical effect but their vibrations influence the psyche of the horse in an energetic way. Therefore they will not excrete any harmful residues, which would justify doping allegations. However, if Rescue Remedy drops are given, the stringent analysis undertaken in laboratories today can detect the alcoholic carrier substance. Up to two days before a competition Rescue Remedy drops should be given in a mixture (10 drops in 20ml of still water). Alternatively the treatment can be given in the form of globules (see page 18).

Sources for purchasing Bach Flowers remedies

The original Bach Flower remedies are produced in England by A. Nelson & Co. and are available in Germany in chemists – either as single flowers in stock bottles or as complete sets. In Austria they are also available individually in pharmacies. In Switzerland they are widely obtainable from a range of chemists and pharmacies.

Leading chemists also sell combinations of flowers, which are ready to take if specifically requested. If it becomes apparent in the course of the therapy that a long-term treatment is necessary, it is advisable to obtain the required flowers as stock bottles.

There are also several sources to be found on the Internet, which offer a variety of ways of obtaining Bach Flower remedies relatively cheaply either as liquid essences or globules. A few selected website addresses have been given in the appendix (see page 107).

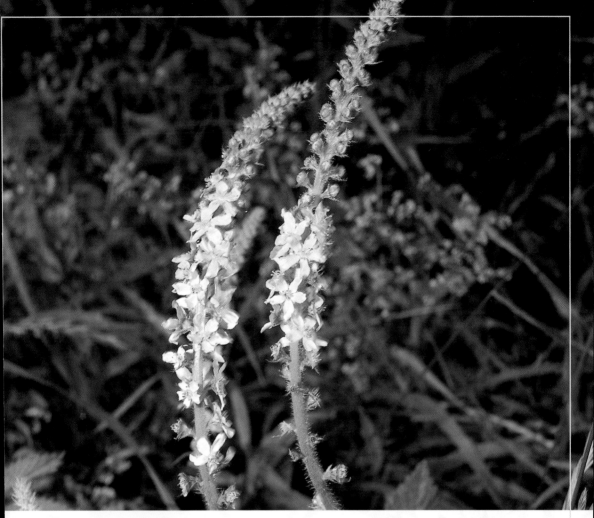

Agrimony — The flower of honesty. Photo: Dr Aichele

The flowers used in Bach Flower remedies

1. Agrimony

Horses that need Agrimony are sociable and peaceful. They seem happy and despite detectable illness are driven to keep active. Calm and peace are important to these animals. If their equilibrium is disturbed they are prone to a great deal of inner conflict and they try to cover up their restlessness.

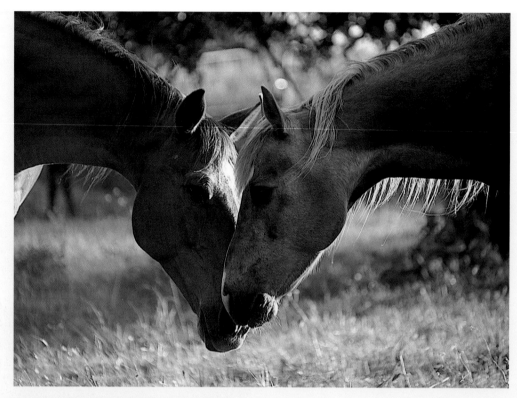

Agrimony-horses desperately need harmony and always greet strange horses with a show of friendliness. Photo: Schmelzer

They are constantly in motion whether with the herd or in their stables. These horses are highly sensitive to everything that disturbs their stability. They bolt down their food, are friendly towards other horses and appear to naturally tolerate being pestered by other horses. Agrimony-horses play down their illness. Even when they are unwell these animals often display an increased need to be active. When being ridden these horses are usually uncomplicated and obedient; however the reverse side of this is that they are easily distracted and lose energy very quickly. This flower also serves to aid detoxification after the horse has been subjected to a physically demanding task, following a long distance ride for example.

Agrimony is the so-called flower of honesty: it enables horses to deal with conflict. In a positive state the horses begin exhibiting signs of happiness once more and give an impression of equilibrium. Agrimony helps to restore inner calm and peace.

Symptoms and uses
- Distraction
- Abscesses
- Fear of being alone
- Problems with adapting
- Lack of stamina
- Easily influenced
- Intense desire to be active

Agrimony

- Problems adjusting following a change of stable or owner
- Sensitivity towards reprimands
- Detoxification (to accompany treatment)
- Peace-loving temperament
- Sensitivity to noise
- Eating with a hearty appetite
- Skin complaints
- Physical overburdening
- Nervousness
- Infected by parasites
- Weaknesses
- Signs of overexertion
- Excess weight
- Indecision
- Lack of peace
- Submissiveness
- Frequent injuries
- Fear of loss
- Gaping wounds (to accompany treatment)
- Caution

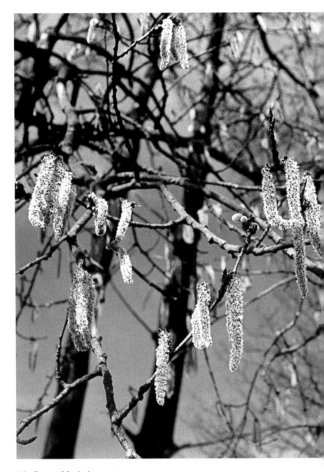

The flower of foreboding – Aspen.
Photo: Institute for Bach Flower Therapy, Andreas Bock

2. Aspen

Aspen-horses are jumpy and sensitive; they are conspicuous for their nervous behaviour. The reasons for this are often unclear; there does not appear to be a good cause for their fear. These animals often have restless sleep patterns, tremble with fear and give the impression of being highly agitated. They will avoid certain places out of fear – these horses often shy away from things, are very sensitive, nervous and extremely delicate. They do not like to be alone and they can become rigid with fear. Aspen is one of the most potent flowers to deal with fear, and it is in marked contrast to the flower Mimulus, which helps with fear of very concrete things. With Aspen we are dealing with confused, inexplicable fear. Nevertheless the two flowers are often combined in a remedy, since horses that need Aspen for fear of unknown things, have often also developed concrete fears of known things. Sensitive Aspen-horses also absorb tension and fear from their rider. The flower is aimed at horses who have been mistreated or those who have suffered from a heightened sensitivity to changes in the weather as well.

Aspen, the flower of foreboding, helps to establish greater courage and trust. In a positive state the

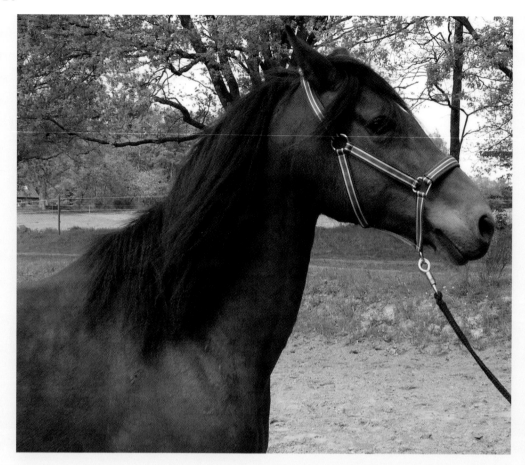

horses are much less intimidated, react in a calmer manner to situations that inspire fear and have more inner confidence and faith.

The Aspen-horse is recognisable through its fundamental nervousness and marked sensitivity. Photo: Bosse

Symptoms and uses

- General fear, inexplicable fear
- Fear in unfamiliar surroundings
- Fear of punishment
- Fear of being alone
- Fear of being touched
- Fear of loud noises such as thunder
- Intestinal problems, bowel problems, diarrhoea (to accompany treatment)
- Sensitivity
- Frantic through fear

- Despondency
- Bad behaviour due to mistreatment
- Change of owner
- Nervousness
- Panic
- Jumpiness
- Excessive sensitivity
- Fear of loud noises and bangs (such as during New Year's Eve celebrations)
- Sensitivity to changes in the weather
- Trembling

Aspen

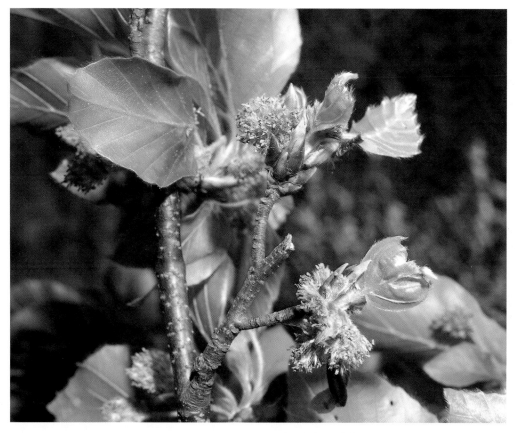

Beech — The flower of tolerance. Photo: Dr. Aichele

3. Beech

Beech-horses are intolerant, often instigate fights or protest most forcefully against something, even directing their behaviour towards the rider. They can become irritated by the tiniest of things and this often leads to aggressive behaviour patterns both towards other horses, who are basically seen as potential foe, and also towards humans. Self-destructive behaviour such as constant kicking at the door of the box or biting their own coat can often ensue. These extremely self-assured animals isolate themselves from the herd and attack any other approaching animals. As a result of their arrogance, constant desire to attack others and their excessive will, they have enormous problems making contact with other horses and cause constant unrest in the herd. Beech is known as the most important flower for dealing with allergies and is successfully used to combat summer eczema sweet itch, food and dust allergies, as well as allergies from insect bites. Beech is also the most suitable flower for dealing with a mother's excessive protectiveness towards her foal and horses that have severe difficulties in adjusting to new situations.

Beech, the flower of tolerance, strengthens the ability to be tolerant. In a positive state these horses have learned to accept other horses and humans and even to greet them in an open and friendly manner. Beech promotes gentleness.

Beech-horses are often aggressive, not only towards other horses and people, but they may also inflict injuries upon themselves by biting for example. Photo: Schmelzer

Symptoms and uses

- Rejection of other horses or people
- Weak immune system
- Aggression
- Inclination to fight
- Difficulty in adjusting
- Tension
- Arrogance
- Arthrosis (to accompany treatment)
- Revolt against other members of the herd or the rider
- Bucking
- Dominance
- Biting its own coat
- Refusing food as a form of protest
- Food allergies (to accompany treatment)
- Problems with joints
- Skin problems
- Difficulty making contact with other members of the herd
- Sensitivity to pain
- Obsession with feuds
- Excessive protectiveness (foals)
- Extreme will
- Instability
- Cantankerousness
- Refusal as a form of protest

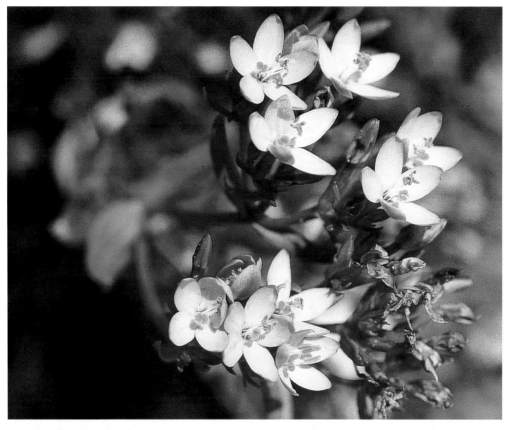

Centaury-The flower of service.
Photo: Institute for Bach Flower Therapy, Andreas Bock

4. Centaury

The essence Centaury is suitable for weak-willed, calm and good-natured horses. They are usually all too well behaved and ready to learn. They may allow their riders to overstretch them until they are totally exhausted. These horses cannot assert themselves, tolerate anything from other horses and occupy a subordinate and passive position within the herd. On the physical side they have an increased susceptibility to infections, attacks by parasites and injuries or wounds. Centaury-horses find it difficult to concentrate and become tired very quickly as they expect too much from themselves.

As the flower of service, Centaury works on weak-willed animals, enabling them to carry out their tasks just as conscientiously as before but from henceforth better able to recognise their own limits and regulate their strength. Centaury promotes vitality and the ability to achieve.

Symptoms and uses
- Difficulty in adjusting to new things
- Respiratory problems
- Chronic illnesses (to accompany treatment)

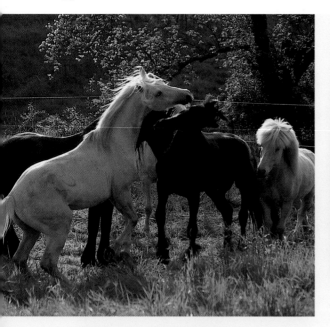

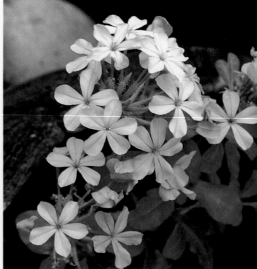

Cerato - The flower of intuition. Photo: IPO

With the support provided by the flower Centaury, the shy horse learns to take an active role in the herd and not to tolerate everything imposed on him by other horses. Photo: Schmelzer.

- Sensitivity to noise and light
- Exhaustion
- Fixation with another horse or owner
- Good natured
- Frequent injuries or illnesses
- Coughing (to accompany treatment)
- Weak immune system
- Feebleness
- Susceptibility to illness
- Frailness
- Compliance
- Passivity
- Timidity
- Weakness
- Lack of confidence
- Uncertainty
- To support the horse while convalescing after an illness
- Submissiveness
- Weak willed

5. Cerato

Cerato-horses are recognisable through their tendency to behave in an unstable and volatile manner. They come across as hesitant and inhibited, often uncertain when in contact with other horses, and they occupy a very lowly position within the herd. They follow unclear signals from anyone at all and not only from the people that look after them. They can also develop an unhealthy dependence on their owner. They become scared if they are left alone, and they appear unsettled and indecisive, as if they are afraid to make a mistake. Young horses, as well as foals that have been separated too early from their mother, need the support provided by this flower most of all.

Cerato is the flower of intuition and helps the horse to have more confidence in its own abilities. In a positive state Cerato-horses shows signs of being curious and eager to learn, they use their own initiative and are less dependent on others. Cerato promotes natural self-confidence.

Centaury

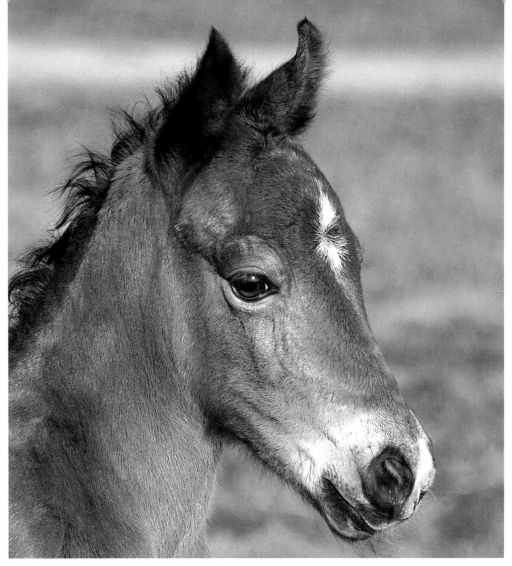

Foals that have been separated from their mother too can early become unstable and volatile. Cerato helps to establish greater self-confidence.
Photo: Schmelzer

Symptoms and uses

- Allergies (to accompany treatment)
- Nervousness
- Fear of being alone
- Problems when mare is being covered, mare does not conceive
- Developmental abnormalities
- Weakness in joints (to accompany treatment)
- Homesickness
- Inhibitions
- Heart problems (to accompany treatment)
- Problems in making contact with other horses
- Concentration problems
- Lack of self-confidence
- Distrust
- Imitation of other members of the herd
- Restlessness
- Indecision
- Lack of independence
- Submissiveness
- Mood swings
- Destructive mania

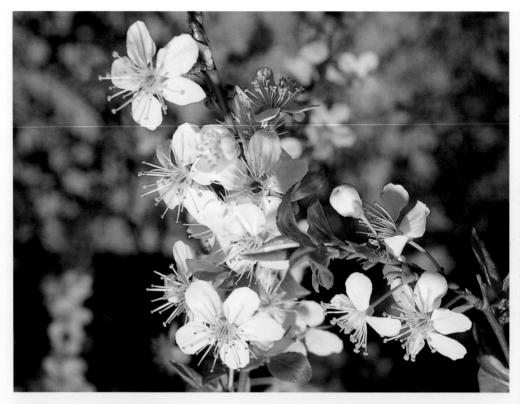

Cherry Plum - The flower of composure. Photo: Dr. Aichele

6. Cherry Plum

Horses that require Cherry Plum are under a great deal of pressure from within and are prone to temperamental outbursts. Suppressed fears can suddenly burst forth in a violent manner: the horses in question "crack up", are unpredictable and can be dangerous in this state. They often come across as volatile or even compulsive. Cherry Plum-horses often have to endure great anguish (for example being transported to the slaughter-house), have not been kept in suitable conditions or have simply been mistreated.

Cherry Plum is the right flower for horses who have had an accident or a similar frightening experience, for mares following a stillbirth as well as for foals who have been separated from their mother too early. Their life force seems diminished and the animals are often strained, highly-strung and tense.

Cherry Plum, the flower of composure, helps to promote inner peace. The horse becomes more balanced and the violent outbursts are not as strong or even disappear altogether.

Symptoms and uses

- Fear
- Aggression towards other horses
- Allergies (to accompany treatment)
- Tension
- Viciousness i.e. during grooming
- Bucking
- Diarrhoea (to accompany treatment)

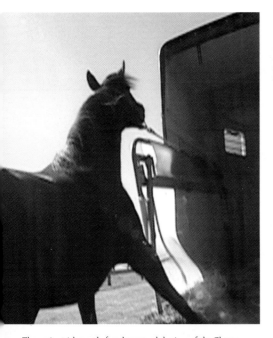

The panic stricken and often dangerous behaviour of the Cherry Plum-horse is frequently a result of traumatic experiences.

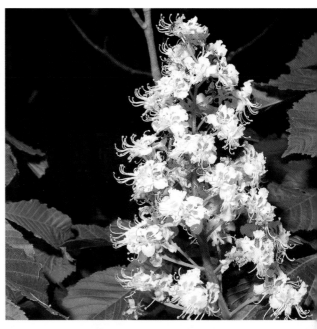

The flower of learning – Chestnut Bud. Photo: Dr. Aichele

- Problems settling in
- Irritability
- Skin disorders (to accompany treatment)
- Colic (to accompany treatment – consult vet!)
- Problems making contact with other horses within the herd
- Muscular tension
- Nervousness
- Jumpiness
- Rearing
- Excessive protectiveness
- Sudden temperamental outbursts
- After traumatic experiences (accident, shock)
- Lack of self control
- Unpredictability
- Inner restlessness
- Problems with the digestive tract (to accompany treatment)
- Trembling with tension and agitation

7. Chestnut Bud

Chestnut Bud-horses always make the same mistakes. They seem unable to learn from past experiences and appear restless and clumsy. It is difficult to teach these horses new skills because of their lack of attentiveness. In addition to this they forget certain manoeuvres even though they are well known to them and have been practiced several times and they seem to shy away from the same hurdles. Chestnut Bud should not be given as a preventive measure to young horses but rather prescribed only in cases of repeated inattentiveness that has not been caused by excessive demands being placed upon them. It is highly characteristic for these horses to be prone to frequently recurring bouts of illnesses such as muscle cramp or respiratory problems. These horses are also prone to injuries because of their foolishness and lack of

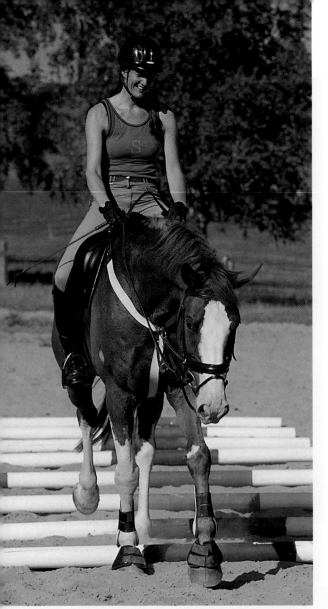

A Chestnut Bud-horse is very inattentive when working, learns very slowly and often makes the same mistakes. Photo: van Damsen

Symptoms and uses

- Distraction
- Allergies (to accompany treatment)
- Fear of new things
- Slowness to grasp new skills
- Chronic illnesses i.e. coughing
  (to accompany treatment)
- Intestinal problems (diarrhoea,
  constipation – to accompany treatment)
- Birthing difficulties
- Weak immune system
- Problems with concentration
- Susceptibility to cramp
- Muscle spasms
- Learning blockages
- Restlessness
- Inattentiveness
- Impatience
- Inability to be taught
- Clumsiness
- Lack of independence
- Lack of care
- Forgetfulness
- Frequent injuries
- Constant repetition of the same mistakes

care. Chestnut Bud is useful for dealing with colic caused by the weather and problems during birth.

Chestnut Bud serves as the flower of learning – it helps concentration and improves the horse's self-awareness. In a positive state these horses visibly make an effort to do everything correctly and conduct themselves with more care and poise.

8. Chicory

Chicory-horses always want to be the centre of attention. They expect the person looking after them to be devoted to them and if this does not happen they will visibly protest to get themselves noticed. They behave in a selfish, obtrusive and demanding manner. They are domineering towards other members of the herd and easily rankled. When they are ill these horses are overcome with self-pity, they have a tendency to exaggerate and mares are

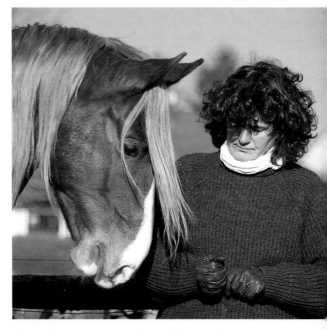

Chicory - The mothering flower. Photo: IPO

The chicory-horse expects to receive the undivided attention of the person looking after it. Photo: Schmelzer

over-attentive to their foals. Many horses appear "offended" if the person that cares for them is absent for a long time. These horses do not generally like to be alone. Chicory is recommended for detoxification and liver problems. It is often used in conjunction with Heather.

The mothering flower, Chicory helps to reverse conditioning and to develop selfless love. In a positive state the obtrusiveness of these horses is greatly reduced and they are more balanced and less dominant.

Symptoms and uses
- Dependence on other horses or carers
- Weak immune system
- Tendency to cling to others
- Obtrusiveness
- Chronic respiratory problems and problems with the digestive tract
- Dominance
- Egotism
- Detoxification, purification (to accompany treatment)
- Demanding behaviour
- Joint complaints
- Domineering behaviour
- Hysteria
- Low immunity
- Moodiness
- Liver problems (to accompany treatment)
- Distrust
- Unforgiving character
- Nervousness
- Irritability
- Stiffness in movements
- Excessive care shown towards mares
- Cantankerousness towards other horses
- Fear of loss
- Self-pitying

Chicory

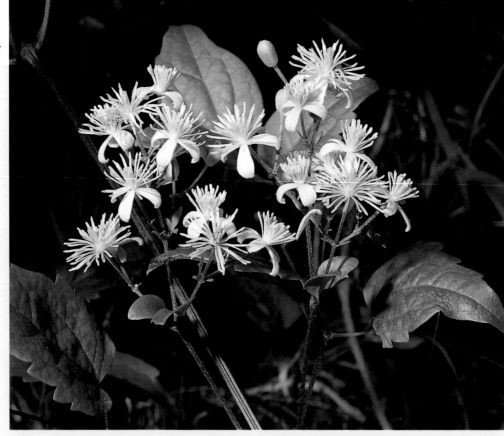

The flower of reality — Clematis.
Photo: Christine Steimer

9. Clematis

Clematis-horses appear dreamy and listless and take little interest in their surroundings. They seem to be present only in the physical sense. It is difficult to motivate them and they project a general lack of interest. They seem to need an extraordinary amount of sleep. In their daily work they are often slow, clumsy and unable to concentrate. This often leads to problems with learning new skills and causes them to come to a standstill in their training. These horses seem to possess a very slender survival instinct and when ill, are often completely apathetic and lack the will to recover.

Clematis is the ideal flower for strengthening the immune system and for detoxification. The flower of reality, it helps horses to cope with the present.

In a positive state they react once more to stimuli like shouting and appear to take a greater interest in their environment. Clematis increases activity and pleasure in life.

Symptoms and uses

- Vacant nature
- Susceptibility to illnesses
- Lack of impetus
- Apathy
- Lack of desire to move
- Disinterest
- Sensitivity to noise
- Indifference

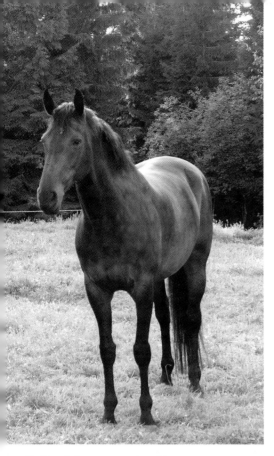

The Clematis-horse appears pensive and dreamy.
He lacks interest in the present. Photo: Bosse

- Weak immune system
- Lack of interest
- Lack of concentration
- Difficulties with learning new things
- Phlegmatic behaviour
- Intense need to sleep
- Overcoming shock after accidents
- Jumpiness
- Sensitivity
- Useful for making the horse stable after being badly treated
- Listlessness
- Lethargy
- Sadness
- Dead to the leg when being ridden
- Clumsiness

10. Crab Apple

Horses who need Crab Apple seem restless and often shy away as if under duress. They are highly susceptible to allergies, infestations by parasites and infectious skin conditions as well as recurring infections. It would be advisable for a vet to examine them to ascertain whether they are actually suffering from some form of illness! Their coat is often dull and not shiny. These horses are very particular and fastidious with regard to different types of food and drinking water. Crab Apple has been used as a follow-up treatment to poisoning and can also be given after medication such as worming treatments and antibiotics.

The cleansing flower, Crab Apple helps horses to accept themselves. In a positive state the organic illnesses and periodic allergies will appear less often. These horses become calmer and stop their persistent nibbling, licking or tendency to shy away. Crab Apple helps to rid the body of poisonous substances or waste products and strengthens the immune system.

Crab Apple - the cleansing flower.
Photo: Institute for Bach Flower Therapy, Andreas Bock

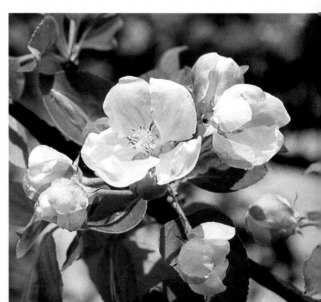

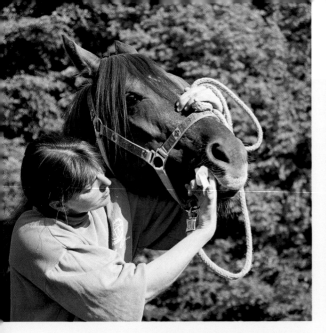

Crab Apple has proved very effective in eliminating poisonous substances and also following worming treatment. Photo: Schmidtke

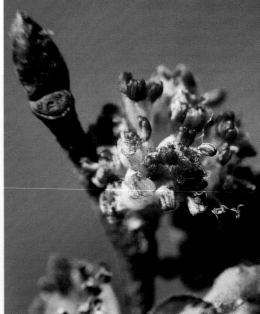

Elm – The flower of responsibility and strength.
Photo: Institute for Bach Flower Therapy, Andreas Bock

Symptoms and uses

- Allergies (to accompany treatment)
- Susceptibility to illnesses
- Fear of puddles
- Following treatment with antibiotics
- Loss of appetite
- Respiratory problems
- Conjunctivitis
- Chronic inflammations and illnesses
- Chronic coughing (to accompany treatment)
- Eczema
- Purification and detoxification (to accompany treatment)
- Skin conditions
- Weak immune system
- Recurring illnesses
- Mite infection
- Restlessness
- Following poisoning of any nature (to accompany treatment)
- Fastidious attitude towards food and drinking water

11. Elm

Elm-horses suffer from severely over-exerting themselves; they often give the impression of being exhausted and despondent. If they are normally full of strength, reliable and ready to work, they now no longer seem able to rise to the challenge. Nervousness and sudden fatigue are characteristic of this state. They react frantically and tensely when carrying out well-known manoeuvres, suddenly refuse simple jumps and appear tired and overburdened. While giving this flower it is important to be able to actually reduce the demands made on the horse! Elm provides a great deal of support in preparation for birth and before big challenges.

Elm, the flower of responsibility and strength, helps to re-establish faith in one's own ability. In a positive state these horses are receptive and accept support when it is given – in terms of no longer having to push themselves to achieve unrealistic goals.

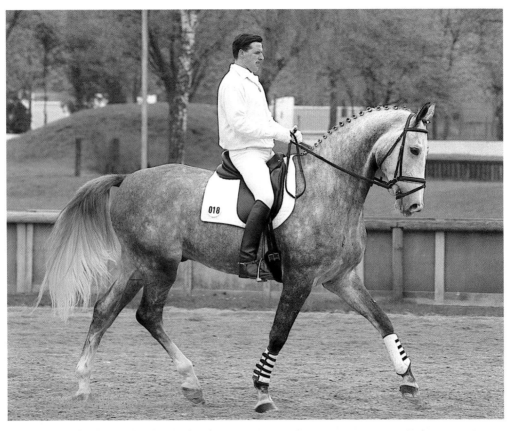

A horse that is normally reliable and readily co-operates with its rider but suddenly seems overburdened, can be helped to find new strength.
Photo: Busch

Symptoms and uses

- Severe illnesses (to accompany treatment)
- Apathy as a result of stress
- Arthritis, arthrosis
- Change of owner
- Permanent stress, strain
- Lack of energy
- Sudden fatigue
- Exhaustion through over-exertion
- Preparation for birth and following difficult births
- Problems with joints
- Infections
- Colic (to accompany treatment – consult vet!)
- Listlessness
- Lack of condition
- Difficulty with concentration
- Lack of strength
- Sudden inability to achieve
- Tiredness
- Nervousness through stress and over-exertion
- Despondency
- Restlessness
- Inner over-exertion
- Uncertainty
- Preparation for competitions

Elm

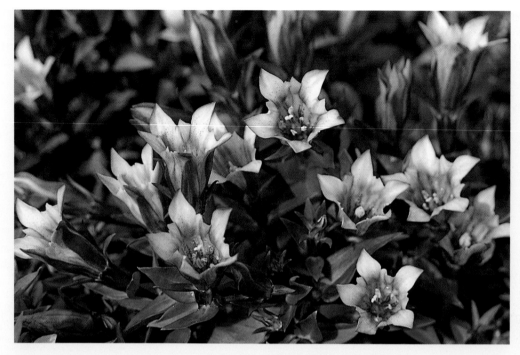

Gentian - The flower of belief. Photo: IPO

12. Gentian

Gentian is the right flower for distrustful, disgruntled horses that are easily discouraged. Their excessive caution and hesitancy causes them to shrink back when touched or at feeding times. They are extremely wary of other horses and of their owners. These symptoms are often caused by a change of stable or owner or even by the loss of a member of the herd in close proximity to them. Most sensitive horses have very little stamina and often absorb insecurities that come from their rider. Gentian is suitable for supporting treatment with long-term illnesses and is often combined with Aspen, Larch and Mimulus.

Gentian, the flower of belief, helps develop courage and optimism. In a positive state the horses lose their fundamental mistrust of everything that is unfamiliar and strange. Gentian increases confidence and calmness.

Symptoms and uses
- Weak immune system
- Fear of new things
- Problems in adjusting
- Apathy
- Agitation in new situations
- Lack of stamina
- Illnesses linked to the auto immune system
  (to accompany treatment)
- Sensitivity to touch
- Change of owner
- Chronic illness and inflammations
  (to accompany treatment)

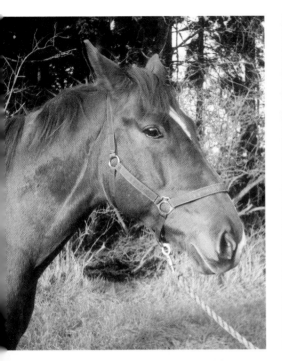

Mistrust is apparent in the horse's expression. Gentian helps to strengthen his courage. Photo: Bosse

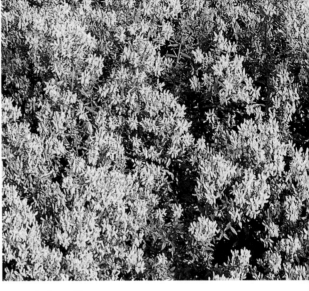

Gorse – the flower of hope.
Photo: IPO

- Chronic coughing (to accompany treatment)
- Lack of endurance
- Propensity towards solitude
- Frailness
- Melancholy
- Mistrust
- Lack of courage
- Despondent character
- Nervousness
- Resignation
- Restlessness
- Limited ability to heal oneself
- Scepticism
- Fear of loud noises, bright lights, sudden bangs
- Uncertainty
- Lack of faith in himself and in others
- Hesitancy

13. Gorse

Gorse is suitable for weak, tired and seemingly resigned horses. They appear apathetic and joyless and it is very difficult to motivate them. Their emotional state is often the result of a long history of suffering and mistreatment. These horses display signs of disturbed behaviour such as wind-sucking or weaving, have a weary look in their eyes and often refuse food. Gorse is used in chronic illnesses in conjunction with Gentian, Hornbeam, Olive and Wild Rose to support the healing of wounds. Gorse is also used in association with Rescue Remedy as a form of euthanasia.

As the flower of hope, Gorse helps horses not to give up altogether and to develop a new will to live. In a positive state, the horses become motivated once again and joy and curiosity reappear.

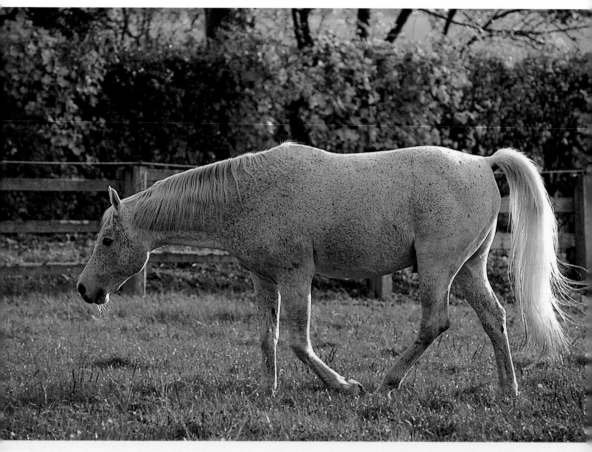

Gorse helps sad and exhausted horses to find new hope and curiosity in life. Photo: van Damsen

Gorse

Symptoms and uses

- Lack of impetus
- Apathy
- Loss of appetite
- Sad, dull expression in eyes
- Chronic inflammations and illnesses (to accompany treatment)
- Exhaustion
- Refusal of food
- Following a long period of suffering, loss or sadness
- Lack of hope
- Reccurring infections
- Lack of interest
- Frailness
- Lethargy
- Lack of enthusiasm
- Tiredness
- Lack of courage
- Lack of motivation
- Despondency
- Resignation
- Giving up on self
- Wounds (to accompany treatment)

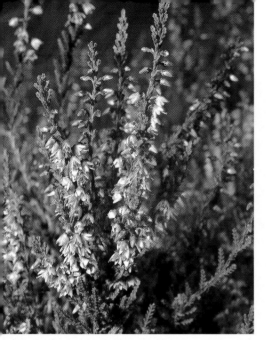

Heather — The flower of identity and independence.
Photo: Dr. Aichele

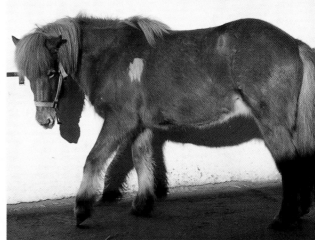

If a Heather-horse is left alone it adopts every possible means to attract attention to itself. Photo: Schmelzer

14. Heather

Heather is suitable for extremely clinging and demanding horses that always want to be the centre of attention. They have a constant need to be near other horses or people and try to get themselves noticed by neighing, scraping, pawing the ground and other forms of behaviour. If a Heather-horse is left alone it will display several bad habits in protest. These animals cling to the stables and to the herd. It is difficult, if not impossible, to get them to ride out unaccompanied. Heather is a very useful when given in preparation for major changes (such as a change of stable or a new herd).

Heather is the flower of identity and independence. It helps with independence and a healthy level of self-confidence. In a positive state horses accept that events do not revolve entirely round themselves. They learn to deal with situations on their own and become more restrained.

Symptoms and uses

- Dependence on owner
- Problems related to old age
- Excessive tendencies to cling
- Loss of appetite
- Obtrusiveness
- Chronic coughing (to accompany treatment)
- Jealousy
- Problems in adapting
- Development of bad habits in order to get noticed
- Illnesses linked to the respiratory tract (to accompany treatment)
- Joint problems (to accompany treatment)
- Clinging behaviour
- Problems making contact with other horses
- Capriciousness
- Unwillingness to learn
- Following a stillbirth
- Healing of scars
- Behaviour as a protest against lack of attention
- Restlessness
- Lack of self-love
- Uncertainty
- Fear of loss
- Self-pity

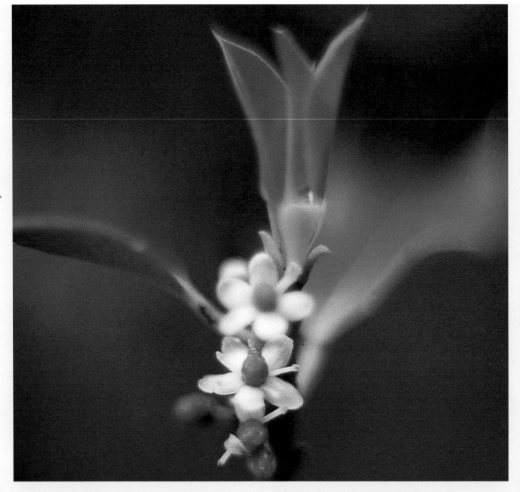

Holly — The flower of the opening of the heart.
Photo: Institute for Bach Flower remedies, Andreas Bock

15. Holly

Holly-horses are jealous and behave in a hostile, angry and aggressive manner. This aggression is usually directed towards a specific horse or person and is caused by jealousy. New members of the herd are rejected and dealt with in a tyrannical way. When in contact with people, the horses kick out and bite and when they are being ridden they express their anger through bucking. Animals that are dissatisfied and not working to their full capacity often display these symptoms. Consequently, the first thing to be done is to change how they are being treated. It is characteristic of these horses to engage in self-destructive behaviour and to have wounds that heal badly.

Holly, the flower of the opening of the heart, helps the horse to know how to deal with negative feelings and to reduce jealousy. In a positive state the horses react in a visibly friendlier manner to those around them. In addition to this they learn how to accept changes in their lives in a calmer manner.

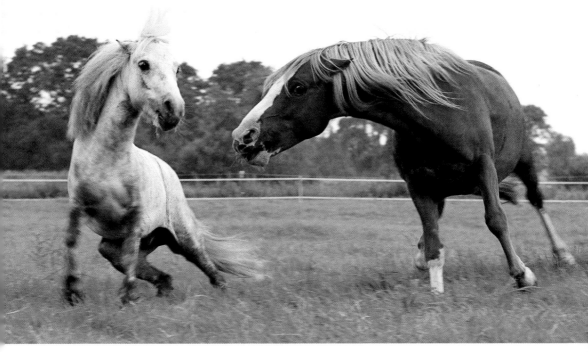

The Holly-horse can be identified by his hostile behaviour towards other members of the herd, wherein he often seeks out a specific victim. Photo:Wedekind

Symptoms and uses

- Negative behaviour
- Aggression, aggressive urge to protect
- Severe illnesses
- Allergies (to accompany treatment)
- Problems related to old age
- Desire to fight
- Arthritis, arthrosis (to accompany treatment)
- Rebelling against the rider
- Biting
- Viciousness
- Bucking
- Dominance
- Diarrhoea (to accompany treatment)
- Bolting
- Jealousy
- Propensity for solitude

- Inflammations (to accompany treatment)
- Agitation
- Hostility towards other horses or people
- Sudden onset of fever
- Colic
- Distrust
- Parasite infestation (to accompany treatment)
- Irritability
- Pains (to accompany treatment)
- Rearing
- Belligerence
- Tyrannical behaviour
- Impatience
- Restlessness
- Refusal to participate in lessons
- Badly healing wounds

Holly

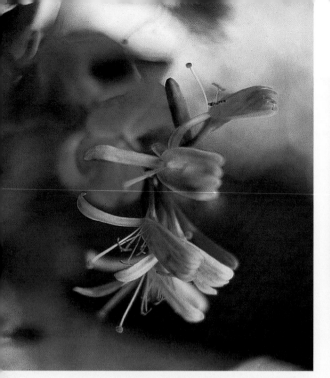

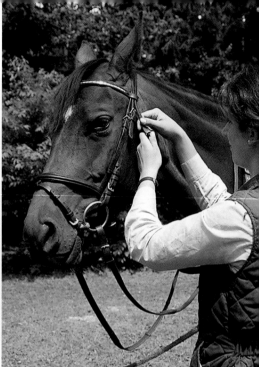

Honeysuckle – the flower of the past.
Photo: Institute for Bach Flower Therapy, Andreas Bock

Honeysuckle-horses appear listless and tolerate everything in a very resigned manner, especially after a traumatic change of stable, yard or owner. Photo: Künzel

16. Honeysuckle

Honeysuckle is the appropriate remedy for listless horses whose behaviour often arises as a result of a change of stable or because of an owner who cannot look after them properly. They take very little notice of their surroundings, refuse food and tasty titbits and visibly suffer at the loss of people or other horses that they have trusted. Sadness and lack of motivation lead to isolation and often to eating disorders. Honeysuckle is suitable to support detoxification and purification. After traumatic experiences it should be given in conjunction with Star of Bethlehem and Walnut. Honeysuckle should also be given to mares before giving birth and to both mares and foals after birth and also during the weaning process in order to ease the transition into their new life. Honeysuckle, the flower of the past, helps horses to process events in the past and strengthens their ability to live in the present with confidence and openness. In a positive state the past is accepted and fades into the background; the horses begin to take an interest in their environment once more and in new things. Honeysuckle increases their pleasure in life.

Symptoms and uses
- Vacant nature
- Problems in adapting
- Lack of impetus
- Apathy
- Change of owner
- No desire to be active
- Problems settling in
- Problems in their relationship to food: food as a substitute or refusal of food due to grief.

- Homesickness
- Infectious illnesses (to accompany treatment)
- Lack of interest
- Problems with concentration
- Circulation problems (to accompany treatment)
- Lack of joy in life
- Melancholy
- Lack of motivation
- Following castration
- Despondency
- New beginnings – following a change
  of stable or owner
- Phlegmatic behaviour
- Resignation
- Listlessness
- Sadness
- Separation from other horses or owner
- Unobservance
- Forgetfulness
- Dreaminess
- Lack of vitality
- Badly healing wounds (to accompany treatment)

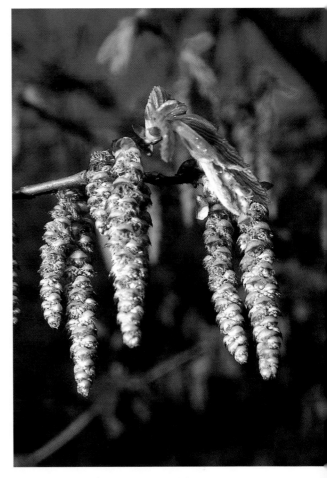

Hornbeam – the flower of vigour. Photo: Dr. Aichele

17. Hornbeam

Horses that require Hornbeam seem tired, weak and unable to concentrate – as though they are overburdened by their duties. They appear to be lacking in motivation and exhausted by the daily routine. However, they approach new challenges with curiosity and enthusiasm. Foals who have developed normally seem to lack strength and energy. Fully-grown horses look completely worn out when the very first symptoms of an illness appear and they take a long time to recover properly. There is a marked tendency towards problems with connective tissue such as reddened conjunctiva. Hornbeam should be used as a follow-up treatment for illnesses and for mental exhaustion, after ruling out the possibility that the horses may actually be overburdened. Hornbeam is especially suitable for weak, old and overloaded animals. Hornbeam, the flower of vigour, promotes verve and vitality. In a positive state, horses are motivated once more and show a new zest for life.

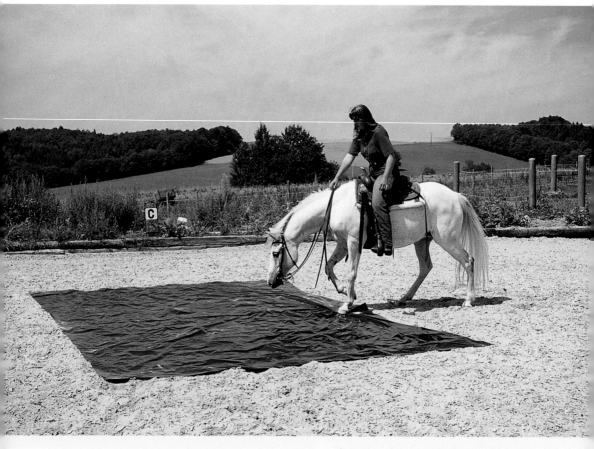

The Hornbeam-horse is typically curious about all new things but remains tired and weak with regard to his daily life. Photo: Ettl

Symptoms and uses

- Allergies (to accompany treatment)
- Problems in old age
- Strain
- Lack of impetus
- Apathy
- Arthritis, arthrosis (to accompany treatment)
- Problems when mare is being covered, mare does not conceive
- Lack of energy
- Exhaustion
- Inappropriate management
- Weak immune system
- Weakness

- Lethargy
- Lack of vitality
- Lack of motivation
- Tiredness
- After a long illness, poor management or overexertion
- Passivity
- Frailty
- Problems with tendons (to accompany treatment)
- Inertia
- Instability
- Boredom if not working to full capacity

Hornbeam

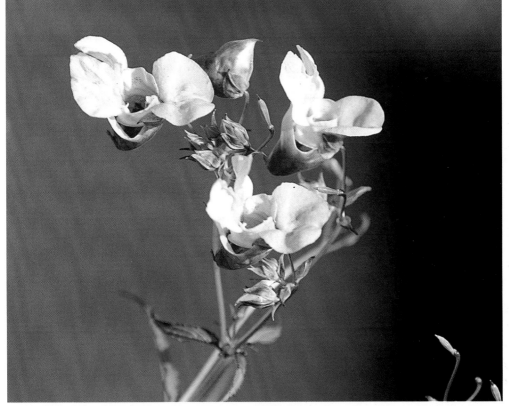

Impatiens — The flower of time. Photo: IPO

18. Impatiens

Impatiens-horses are recognisable through their impatience, frantic nature and irritability. They frequently react exuberantly but at times this can also turn to aggression. They are permanently wired, cannot wait for things and push themselves forward. Competition horses are extremely impatient while performing and have a tendency to make careless mistakes as a result of their hectic pace and lack of focus. They tire very quickly and sweat profusely because of their inner tension. Before giving a Bach Flower remedy it would be important ask a vet to check their thyroid gland as well as to review the way they are managed.

Impatiens, the flower of time, helps to reduce stress and impatience and to develop a sense of calm. In a positive state the horses learn to restrain themselves and become visibly more peaceful and relaxed.

Symptoms and uses
- Aggression as a result of impatience
- Allergies (to accompany treatment)
- Strain
- Quick tempered
- Strong impulse to be active
- Tendency to bite
- Difficulties settling in
- Tendency towards solitude
- Fever
- Food allergies
- Irritability
- Skin problems
- Frantic behaviour
- Heart problems
- Hyperactivity
- Impulsiveness
- Intolerance as a result of impatience

Impatiens

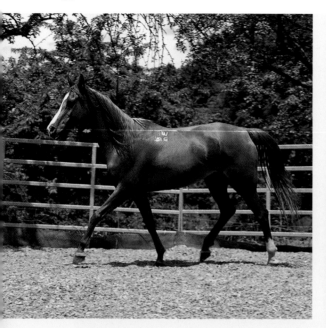

The Impatiens-horse is nervous and tense and seldom at peace.
Photo: Schmelzer

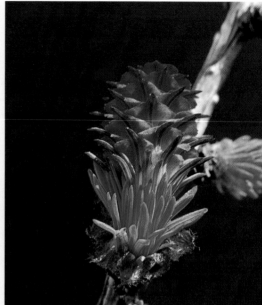

Larch – The flower of self-confidence.
Photo: Institute for Bach Flower Therapy, Andreas Bock

- Colic (to accompany treatment)
- Lack of concentration as a result of impatience
- Capriciousness
- Nervousness
- Irritability
- Carelessness
- Agitation
- Sudden pains
- Tires quickly due to self-imposed over-exertion and restlessness
- Temperamental behaviour
- Instability
- Impatience
- Extreme restlessness
- Problems relating to digestive tract (to accompany treatment)
- Tension
- Grinding of teeth

19. Larch

Larch-horses have very little self-confidence and subordinate themselves to other members of the herd. If other horses challenge these over-cautious and uncertain animals, they retreat immediately. They are hesitant or passive in new and unfamiliar situations. At feeding time they always allow other members of the herd to go before them. They isolate themselves and walk around with both head and tail hanging down. Larch is often recommended for use with Centaury. Larch is the flower to choose to strengthen the immune system. Larch, the flower of self-confidence, increases faith in one's own abilities and helps to promote self-assurance. In a positive state, the horses lose their wariness of new things and become braver and more stable.

Impatiens

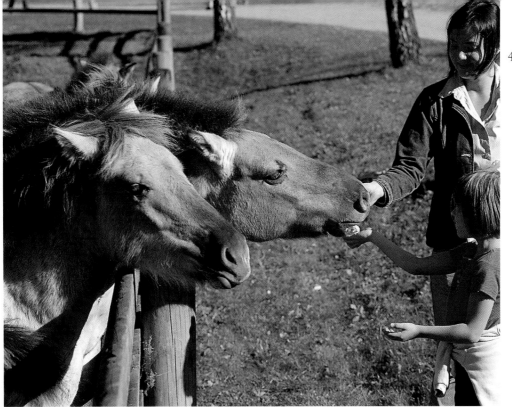

A horse lacking in self-confidence gains in courage as a result of the support provided by Larch.

Symptoms and uses

- Weak immune system
- Fear of new things
- Difficulties in adjusting
- Lack of impetus
- Apathy
- Lack of stamina
- Lack of achievement compared to other horses
- Sensitivity
- Obsession with food as a substitute
- Skin problems (to accompany treatment)
- Helplessness
- Difficulties making contact with other horses
- Susceptibility to illness
- Frailness
- Distrust
- Despondency
- Compliance

- Reserve
- Resignation
- Shyness
- Fragility
- Lack of self-confidence
- Sensibility
- Clumsiness
- Uncertainty
- Submissiveness
- Excessively cautious
- Hesitancy

Larch

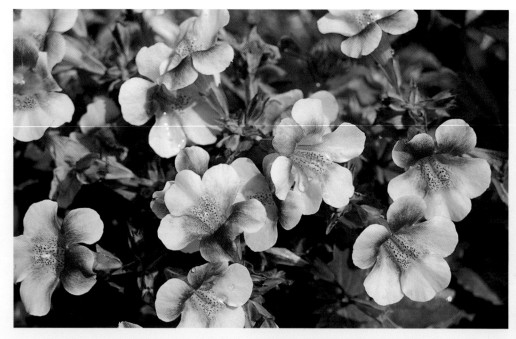

Mimulus — the flower of bravery. Photo: IPO

20. Mimulus

Mimulus is the ideal flower for shy, anxious horses that often react in an oversensitive manner or display a fear of specific situations. They are guarded and nervous and seem to be afraid of other horses, people or concrete things. Stimuli like sudden noises, movements or light frighten them enormously. If these horses suffer from completely understandable fears, such as being frightened of the farrier and vet, of dogs, horse trailers, water and of being alone, it indicates that Mimulus will be a successful remedy. Changes in their normal environment can frighten these horses long after the event. The horses frequently look to their owner for protection. During a period of convalescence they are very careful and take things easy for a long time – in the case of lameness, for example, the problem will persist even though the original injury is completely healed. Mimulus primarily provides support after injuries and operations.

Mimulus, the flower of bravery, helps to develop courage, to overcome fears and subsequently eliminate them. In a positive state, these horses are less frightened when they are confronted by fear-inducing situations and they show more courage.

Symptoms and uses
- Allergies (to accompany treatment)
- Susceptibility to illness
- Fear of specific things (noises, vet, farrier, being loaded into horse boxes, storms)
- Fear of being alone
- Strain

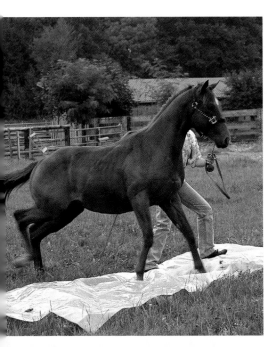

Mimulus helps nervous horses to deal with fear-inducing situations in a considerably more relaxed manner. Photo: Ettl

21. Mustard

Mustard is the appropriate flower for horses that suddenly appear despondent, unenthusiastic and sad for no apparent reason. These animals barely take any notice of their surroundings and show no interest in things that they previously enjoyed. They behave as if they are paralysed and in certain cases even start refusing food. This situation can be turned around again just as quickly as it arose – this periodic appearance of despondency is characteristic of the need for Mustard. The symptoms can often lead owners to wonder whether the horse has been poisoned and a vet should be called immediately to investigate any possible physical causes!

Mustard, the flower of light, helps these horses to enrich their life experience. In a positive state the horses display a much more stable frame of mind and develop a new zest for life.

- Sensitivity to noise and light
- Timorousness
- Skin problems (to accompany treatment)
- Heart problems (to accompany treatment)
- Difficulties making contact with other horses
- Lack of concentration
- Distrust
- Nervousness
- Sensitivity to pain
- Jumpiness
- Sensitivity
- Fear of loud noises, sudden bangs and bright, flashing lights
- Restlessness
- Reserve

Mustard – The flower of light. Photo: IPO

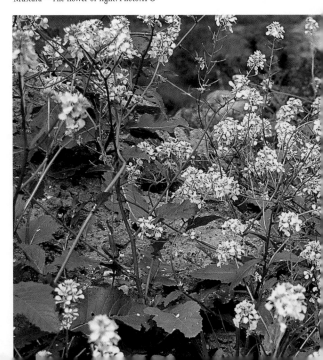

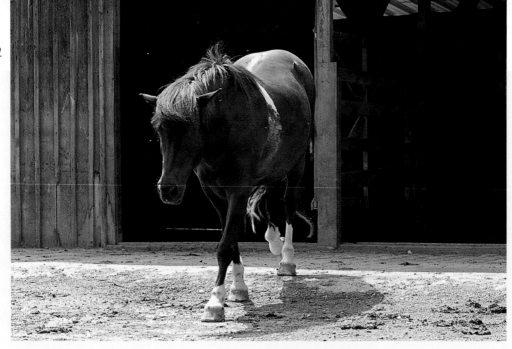

A horse that is despondent and unenthusiastic one moment and then happy again the next, requires the Bach Flower remedy Mustard.
Photo: van Damsen

Symptoms and uses

- Susceptibility to illnesses
- Lack of impetus
- Apathy
- Lack of appetite
- Change of owner
- No desire to be active
- Biting of coat
- Heart problems (to accompany treatment)
- Indifference
- Difficulties making contact with other horses
- Frailness
- Capriciousness
- Listlessness
- Lack of motivation
- Despondency
- Passivity
- Unresponsiveness
- Self-destructive behaviour
- Volatile mood changes
- Inertia
- Lack of vitality

22. Oak

Oak-horses are conscientious, tenacious and ambitious animals. However, they tend to be unaware of their own limitations and carry on working beyond the point of exhaustion. It is clearly apparent that

Oak – The flower of stamina. Photo: Dr.Aichele

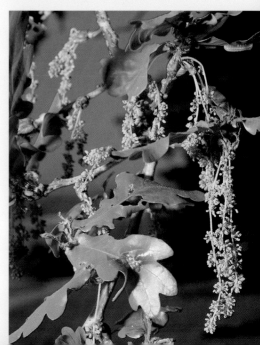

Mustard

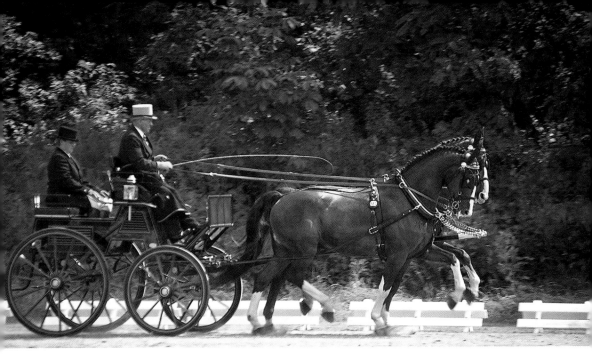

Oak-horses always co-operate with enthusiasm and have a tendency to over-exert themselves.
Photo: Schmelzer

these horses push themselves to such an extent that they cause a great deal of inner strain. Competition and working horses in particular run the risk of overtaxing themselves to the point of total exhaustion. Within the framework of treatment, it is important to rule out the possibility that these horses are actually being over-stretched. Oak is an important flower for easing the transition into life as a retired horse.

Oak, the flower of stamina, helps horses to develop the ability to enjoy life and to relax. In a positive state, the horses reveal a more appropriate level of perseverance. They react normally and become exhausted when placed under excessive strain and thereby learn to pace themselves more realistically.

Symptoms and uses
- Difficulties related to old age
- Strain
- Arthritis, arthrosis (to accompany treatment)
- No desire to be active due to tension or a strong desire to be active
- Chronic illnesses
- Obstinacy
- Ambition
- Coughing (to accompany treatment)
- Hyperactivity
- Ignoring exhaustion
- Physical overexertion
- Weakness
- Boredom
- Capriciousness in old age
- Wasting of muscles
- Muscle tension
- Following overtaxing
- Nervousness
- Resignation
- Lively temperament
- Tension
- Breakdown due to over exertion

Oak

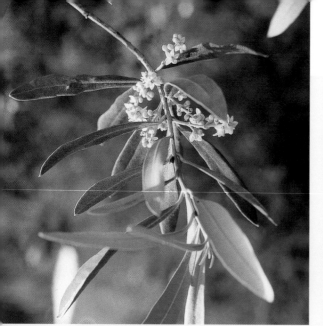

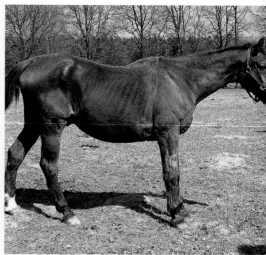

Olive – The flower of revitalisation.
Photo: Institute for Bach Flower Therapy, Andreas Bock

An Olive-horse can be recognised by its poor general state of health and its total exhaustion. Photo: Bolze

23. Olive

Horses who need Olive give the impression of being completely exhausted and devoid of energy; they are extremely tired and lacking in strength and cannot be roused to take part in any activity. They often refuse food or eat without enthusiasm. It seems as if they have completely over-exerted themselves, have been over-stretched or have just recovered from a long illness. Olive is used with older animals and is ideal as an accompanying therapy during illness to improve the general state of health.

Olive, the flower of revitalisation, helps to create new energy in the body. In a positive state, the horses begin to take an interest in life again; they are more easily motivated and develop new vitality.

Symptoms and uses

- Weak immune system
- Following treatment with antibiotics
- Lack of impetus
- Apathy
- Loss of appetite
- Respiratory illnesses
- No desire to be active
- Chronic illnesses
- Problems when mare is being covered
- Lack of energy
- Exhaustion
- Feverish when weak
- To provide support at birth
- Low immunity
- Frailness
- Following a long illness
- Before and after operations
- Resignation
- Weakness
- Complete overexertion

Olive

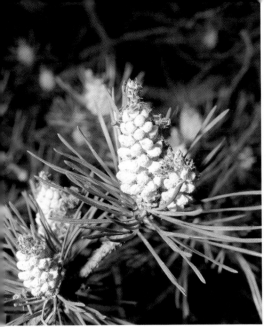

Pine – The flower of self-acceptance and independence.
Photo: Dr. Aichele

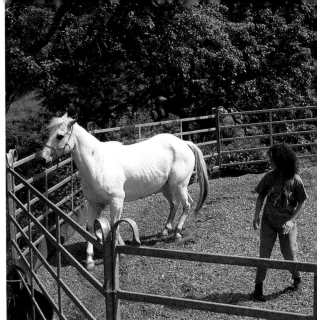

The Pine-horse does not react to clear signals and is fundamentally shy and submissive. Photo: Schmelzer

24. Pine

Pine is suitable for horses that appear despondent and dejected and who are especially sensitive to reprimands. They are conspicuous for the helpless expression in their eyes as well as for their nervous posture, which verges on submissiveness. These horses almost seem to expect to be punished. They often flinch without cause and react in an excessively sensitive manner to being told off and seem to want to withdraw completely. In the hierarchy of the herd, these horses occupy a very lowly position in relation to other horses. Pine is the right choice of flower for horses who have had bad experiences with people or other horses.

Pine, the flower of self-acceptance and independence helps to develop autonomy and to reduce feelings of guilt and dejection. In a positive state, the horses gain in self-confidence without losing their intrinsically cautious nature.

Symptoms and uses
- Allergies
- Fear
- Strain
- Arthritis, arthrosis (to accompany treatment)
- Sensitivity
- State of exhaustion
- Cowardice
- Cringing posture
- Helplessness
- Dejection
- After bad experiences with people or other horses
- Apparent "guilty conscience"
- Timidity
- Jumpiness
- Shyness
- Lack of self love
- Lack of self-confidence
- Uncertainty
- Submissiveness
- Excessive caution

Pine

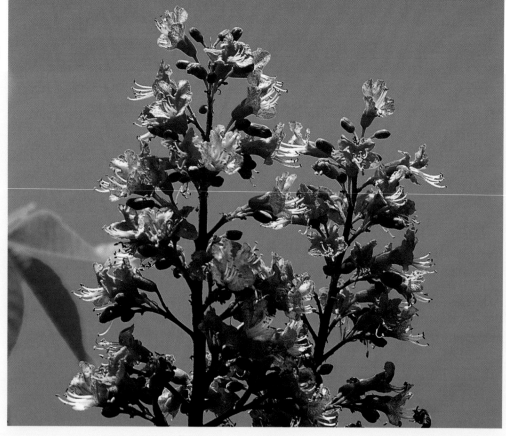

Red Chestnut - The flower of independence and composure.
Photo: IPO

25. Red Chestnut

Horses that try to protect other horses or people in an exaggerated manner can be effectively treated with Red Chestnut. If their owner or a member of the herd with whom they enjoy a particular closeness is absent, these horses become extremely restless and agitated. They often begin to refuse food and seem completely aimless. They will not let anyone near the partner they are protecting (whether it is their owner, foal or other members of the herd) and can even become quite aggressive about it. Stallions or rigs defend their mares to an excessive degree. Red Chestnut is a very important flower in dealing with horses exhibiting extreme concern about their own foals or in the case of a phantom pregnancy. It is also extremely effective in situations involving a change of stable or owner.

It is imperative to distinguish it from the flower, Holly, which focuses on jealousy.

Red Chestnut is the flower of independence and composure. It helps to lessen concern for others and to reduce it to a more natural level. In a positive state the horses no longer perceive danger in every stranger and develop trust.

Symptoms and uses

- Dependence on owner or other horses
- Aggression
- Fear of being alone
- Tendency to cling
- Biting
- Sensitivity

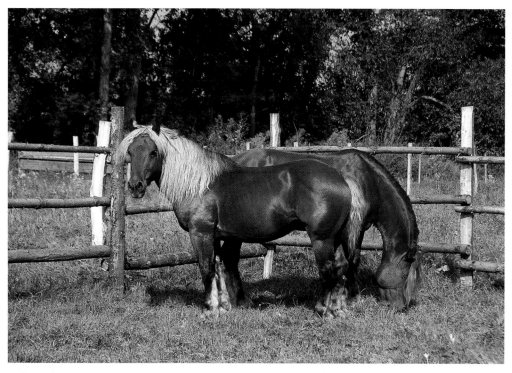

A horse that constantly protects other horses from the herd can reach a calmer state with the help of Red Chestnut. Photo: Schmelzer

26. Rock Rose

- Exhaustion
- Eating disorders: ranging from eating too greedily to refusing food in the event of separation
- Heart problems (to accompany treatment)
- Nervousness
- Agitation
- Phantom pregnancy
- Over zealous leader of the herd
- Excessive care (foals)
- Restlessness

Rock Rose is the right flower for horses that panic easily or suffer from acute fear. They look as if they have lost their senses and seem unaware of their environment. Sheer terror causes them to behave as if they are paralysed and they storm around in wild panic. When they are being ridden these horses are often unpredictable and have a tendency to bolt, rear, buck or lash out as soon as they are gripped by fear. They often suffer from diarrhoea caused by nerves and as a result of their frantic nature, and from frequent injuries, which are usually self-inflicted. Rock Rose is used for severe nervous conditions (for example during storms or firework celebrations) and also in life-threatening situations such as before an operation or after giving birth, after colic, accidents or mistreatment. The flower can also be

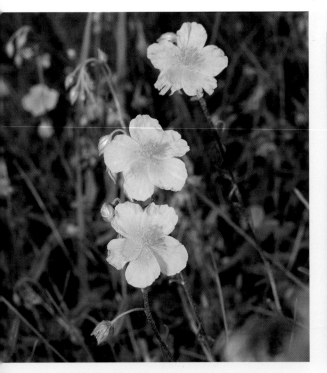

Rock Rose - The flower of escalation. Photo: Dr. Aichele

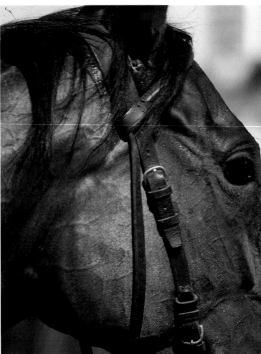

Consumed with fear and attempting to escape: Rock Rose is advisable for situations like these. Photo: Schmelzer

used as an accompanying treatment after heatstroke, sunburn, unconsciousness and allergic shock.

Rock Rose, the flower of escalation, helps the horse to keep calm and take courage when he is panicking. In a positive state, the horses learn how to cope with similarly loaded situations that may reoccur. They also develop courage to deal with life.

Symptoms and uses
- Aggression due to fear
- Acute fear and panic
- Allergic shock (to accompany treatment)
- Fear of being held tight or tethered
- Bleeding (to accompany treatment)
- Biting due to fear
- Disturbance of consciousness (to accompany treatment)
- Diarrhoea (to accompany treatment)
- Bolting due to panic
- Tendency to escape
- Fear of storms
- Heatstroke
- Hysteria
- Paralysis due to panic
- After insect bites, accidents or shock
- Sunstroke
- Fear of loud noises, sudden bangs and bright flashing lights
- Rigidity due to panic
- Hypothermia
- Trembling

Rock Rose

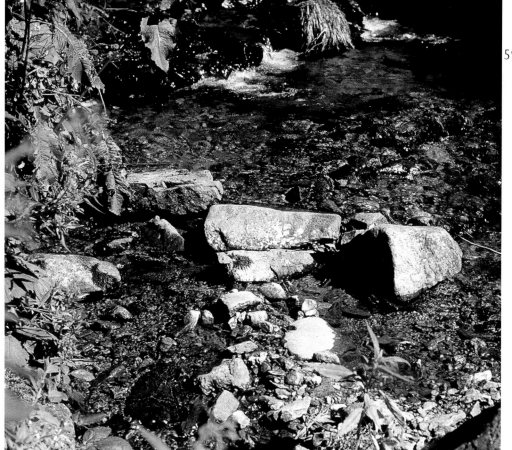

Rock Water – The flower of flexibility.
Photo: Institute for Bach Flower Therapy, Andreas Bock

27. Rock Water

The essence, Rock Water, is suitable for horses that suppress their own fundamental needs in favour of a harsh discipline. They seem to be permanently at the peak of fitness and show great determination. Their inner tension reveals itself in stiff, awkward movements. These horses have very distinct characteristics and they react to any changes in their lives with signs of stress such as a dull coat. Mares create problems when being covered and have difficulty in conceiving.

Rock Water has proved to be very effective in treating constipation, stiff joints, arthritis, arthrosis and cramp.

Rock Water, the flower of flexibility, helps to promote a zest for life and openness in relation to the environment of horses. In a positive state, the horses relax; they become more open to their surroundings and no longer seem to be so self-obsessed. The horses discover new agility and ease.

Symptoms and uses

- Allergies (to accompany treatment)
- Strain
- Arthritis, arthrosis (to accompany treatment)
- Sensitivity to touch
- Problems when mare is being covered, mare does not conceive
- Tendency to solitude
- Eating disorders
- Homesickness

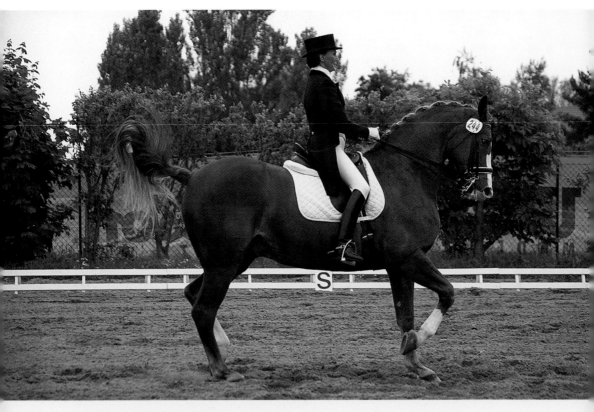

Horses that require the essence Rock Water deny their own needs and often appear very tense. Photo: Schmelzer

Rock Water

- Coughing (to accompany treatment)
- Self - intolerance
- Problems making contact with other horses
- Cramps (to accompany treatment)
- Muscular tension
- Nervousness
- Stubbornness
- Stiffness
- Inability to concentrate
- Inflexibility
- Restlessness
- Determination
- Illnesses linked to the digestive tract (to accompany treatment)
- Constipation (to accompany treatment)

28. Scleranthus

Scleranthus-horses are distinctive due to their instability, frantic reactions and generally volatile behaviour. They have little stamina, are easily distracted and have difficulties in concentrating. These horses are generally regarded as unreliable and moody. Typical symptoms include a varying appetite, impaired balance, fluctuating temperature and a tendency to alternate between having constipation and diarrhoea. Scleranthus is also effective in dealing with skin problems and sensitivity to changes in the weather.

Scleranthus, the flower of balance, helps to create greater flexibility with regard to changes in the environment of horses and inner harmony.

In a positive state, the horses appear less volatile and become more decisive and adaptable.

Symptoms and uses

- Easily distracted
- Allergies (to accompany treatment)
- Loss of appetite
- Respiratory problems (to accompany treatment)
- Lack of stamina
- Alternating diarrhoea and constipation
- Eating disorders (to accompany treatment)
- Impaired balance
- Skin conditions
- Frantic nature
- Hyperactivity
- Colic following changes in the weather
- Problems with concentration
- Circulation problems (to accompany treatment)
- Frailness
- Capriciousness
- Nervousness
- Irritability
- Volatility
- Fluctuating moods
- Inattentiveness
- Instability
- Changeability
- Indecision
- Restlessness
- Uncertainty
- Sensitivity to changes in the weather
- Badly healing wounds (to accompany treatment)

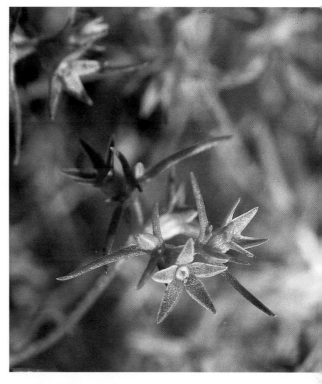

Scleranthus – The flower of balance.
Photo: Institute for Bach Flower Therapy, Andreas Bock

Easily distracted and not at all focused on the task in hand. Scleranthus can help to increase consistency and powers of concentration. Photo: Schmelzer

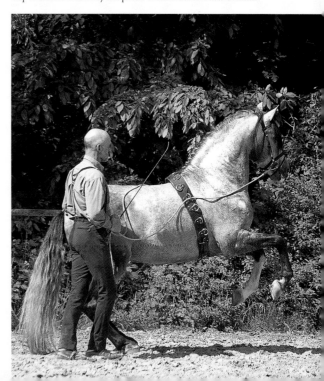

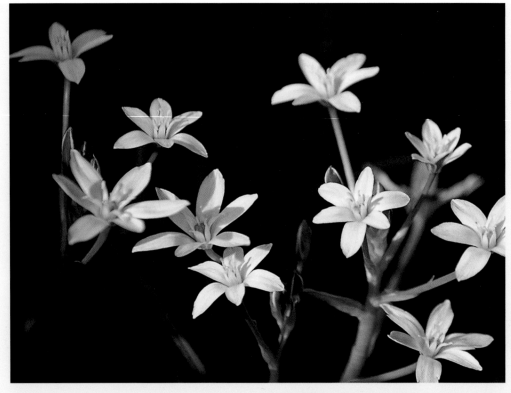

Star of Bethlehem – The flower of comfort. Photo: IPO

29. Star of Bethlehem

Star of Bethlehem is suitable for horses that seem depressed or sad, who have been physically or emotionally shattered (for example as the result of an accident or a change of stable or owner) and who are having difficulties in coming to terms with the experience. These animals appear apathetic and listless. In certain cases the traumatic experience at the heart of the problem can go back a long way, even as far back as birth. Star of Bethlehem serves as a source of comfort for the soul for horses that feel abandoned and unloved. It is the ideal flower to give following a birth or a stillbirth, as well as after a horse has been separated from animals or people with whom they have been in close proximity. Star of Bethlehem is almost always to be found in an initial Bach Flower remedy.

Star of Bethlehem, the flower of comfort helps to get rid of blockages that have been caused by a physical or emotional shock. In a positive state, the horses can come to terms with bad past experiences and deal much better with situations that bring back unpleasant memories.

Symptoms and uses
- Aggression due to distrust
- Allergies (to accompany treatment)
- Fear of known things and situations
- Fear as a result of a shock or trauma

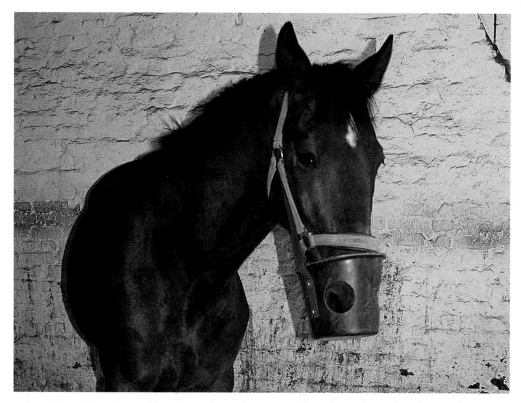

As the flower of comfort, Star of Bethlehem is also effective when given to horses with colic, to reduce the shock. Photo: Bolze

- Lack of impetus
- Apathy
- Loss of appetite due to sadness
- Respiratory illnesses (to accompany treatment)
- Change of owner
- Chronic illnesses (to accompany treatment)
- Diarrhoea (to accompany treatment)
- First thing to be given after an accident
- Extreme fears
- Refusal of food
- Shock at birth (foals and mares)
- Homesickness
- Hopelessness
- Hysteria as the result of shock

- Difficulties making contact with other horses
- Sorrow
- Distrust
- Lack of motivation
- Muscle tension
- Nervousness
- Resignation
- Timidity
- Shock
- Self surrender
- Sadness
- Pain as a result of separation
- Overcoming loss

Star of Bethlehem

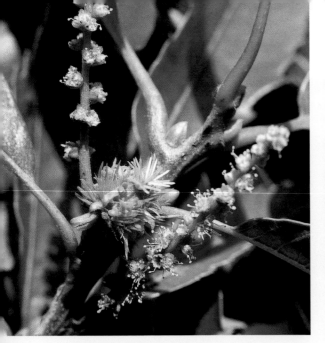

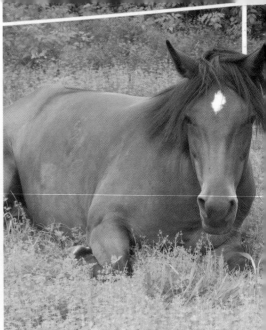

Sweet Chestnut — The flower of release.
Photo: Institute for Bach Flower Therapy, Andreas Bock

Sweet Chestnut can help a weak and exhausted horse to put his despair behind him. Photo: Bosse

30. Sweet Chestnut

Horses that need Sweet Chestnut suffer from inner hopelessness and extreme strain. They are exhausted and no longer take any interest in their environment. These horses isolate themselves, have a very meagre appetite, a dull look in their eyes and apparently no more energy. These symptoms are typical of horses who have been kept in their stables for excessive periods or who have been ill for a long time. The management of these horses should be checked and the demands made on them reduced.

Sweet Chestnut, the flower of relief, helps with depression, inner hopelessness and despair. In a positive state, the horses can be motivated once more; they allow people to help them out of their dejection and are ready to emerge from their despondency and "black cloud". Sweet Chestnut helps increase vitality.

Symptoms and uses

- Fear
- Lack of impetus
- Apathy
- Loss of appetite
- Hopelessness
- Change of owner
- Chronic illnesses (to accompany treatment)
- Exhaustion
- Refusal of food
- Despair
- Loss of interest
- Isolation
- Weakness
- Despondency
- Passivity
- Resignation
- Listlessness
- Sadness
- Disturbed state
- Inner restlessness
- Physical breakdown

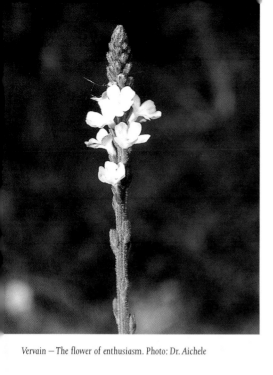

Vervain — The flower of enthusiasm. Photo: Dr. Aichele

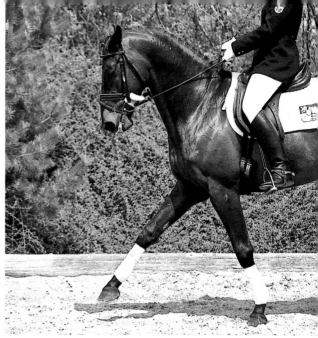

The Vervain-horse cannot conserve his energy and over-exerts himself through his extreme ambition. Photo: Busch

31. Vervain

Vervain is suitable for horses that are hyperactive and become enthusiastic very quickly. They struggle to pace themselves adequately and seemingly never get tired. They are bubbling over with energy and appear to be very determined – until they reach a point of total exhaustion through their own over-exertion. A typical recipient of treatment with Vervain is the leader of the herd who can become aggressive if he is unable to motivate the rest of the herd to follow his wishes. Vervain has been used highly effectively with competition horses that have developed bad habits or quirks. While investigating the reasons behind this behaviour a vet should check both the metabolism and thyroid gland. Vervain is also used for muscular tension, colic caused by cramp and as preparation for birth.

Vervain, the flower of enthusiasm, helps horses to relax and to contain their excessive zeal. In a positive state, calm is visibly restored once more to these hectic horses.

Symptoms and uses

- Aggression
- Problems in adjusting
- Strain
- Brashness
- Seemingly inexhaustible stamina
- Excessive capacity for enthusiasm
- Biting
- Bucking
- Obstinacy
- Dominance
- Strong powers of endurance
- Propensity for solitude
- Sensitivity to reprimands

- Excitability
- Irritability
- Hyperactivity
- Impulsiveness
- Intolerance
- Colic (to accompany treatment)
- Muscular tension (to accompany treatment)
- Nervousness
- Restlessness
- Rearing
- Lively temperament
- Tension
- Wilfulness

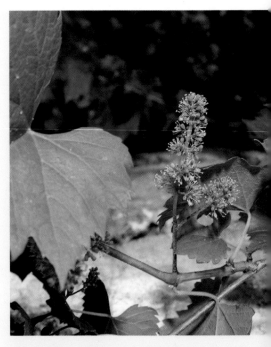

Vine — The flower of authority. Photo: Dr. Aichele

32. Vine

Vine-horses are excessively ambitious and dominant. They tyrannise other members of the herd or even people. Their physical stance conveys their sense of superiority and pride. Within the herd they want to hold a leading position; they are prepared to fight for this and often become loners. They are very difficult to teach due to their obstinacy and refusal to obey commands and they appear very overbearing. Obsessive neuroses such as wind-sucking and weaving are very common. Vine is used as an accompanying treatment for severe chronic illnesses, frequently combined with Heather and Holly.

Vine, the flower of authority, reduces ambition and dominance to normal levels. In a positive state, Vine increases these horses' ability to accept other horses and people and their willingness to be more subordinate.

Symptoms and uses
- Aggression
- Tension
- Obtrusiveness
- Rebelliousness against demanded obedience
- Biting
- Bucking
- Dominance
- Jealousy
- Propensity for solitude
- Hostility
- Imperious behaviour
- Refusal to obey
- Domineeringness
- Intolerance
- Problems making contact with other horses
- Leader of the herd
- Difficulties with learning

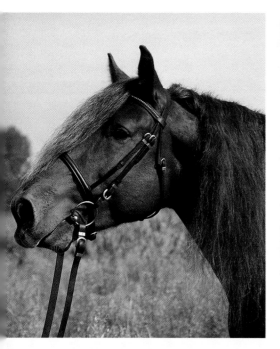

The Vine-horse is full of self-confidence and is very domineering towards people and other horses. Photo: Schmelzer

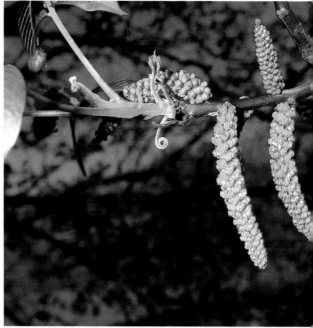

Walnut – The flower of birth. Photo: Dr. Aichele

- Power struggles with riders and other members of the herd
- Muscular tension (to accompany treatment)
- Struggles to establish rank
- Irritability
- Carelessness
- Excessive self-confidence
- Belligerence
- Tyrannical behaviour

33. Walnut

Walnut-horses are very uncertain. They lack direction in their lives and changes of any kind cause them to become highly irritable. They react very sensitively to changes of any kind with a show of bad habits or by becoming ill. Problems can be caused by such things as a new stable or owner, a shift in seasons, or their changing coat. These horses often experience difficulties when they become pregnant, after birth (both mares and foals) or after castration. Walnut is an important flower for older horses whose abilities are waning and is otherwise recommended to ease the transition process with euthanasia. It is usually successful when combined with Honeysuckle.

Walnut, the flower of birth, helps horses to respond to new beginnings in a calm manner and to accept new things. In a positive state, these

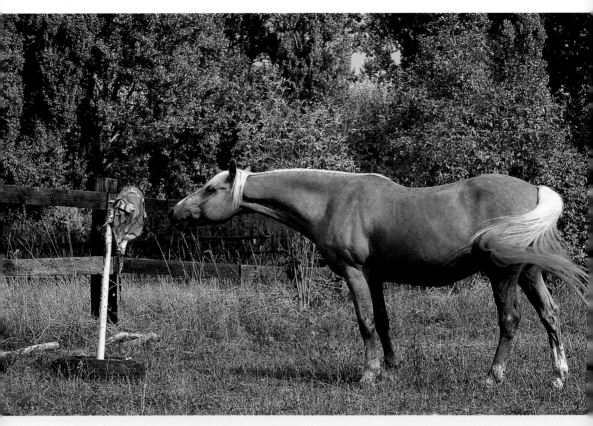

Walnut- horses are characterised by their fear of all new things and a general air of uncertainty. Photo: Schmelzer

horses learn to cope with changes in their lifestyle and visibly react more calmly. Walnut helps increase stability in new situations.

Symptoms and uses

- Changes in circumstances
- Allergies (to accompany treatment)
- Fear of new things
- Fear as a result of stress
- Problems in adjusting
- Loss of appetite
- Lack of stamina and competence
- Change of owner
- Problems settling in
- Refusal of food
- Birth (for mares and foals)
- Homesickness
- Susceptibility to illness
- Frailness
- Change of stable
- Euthanasia
- Susceptibility to stress
- Separation of mares and foals
- Over-sensitivity
- Transition to a new phase of life
- Uncertainty
- Self-pity

Walnut

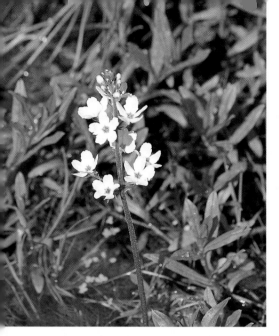

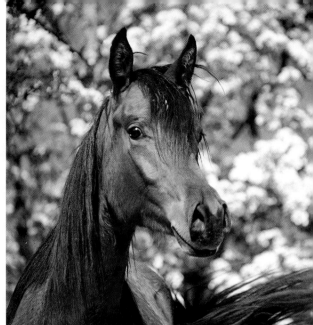

Water Violet – The flower of communication.
Photo: IPO

The Water Violet horse seems proud and unapproachable.
Photo: Schmelzer

34. Water Violet

Water Violet is the appropriate flower for intelligent and proud horses that distance themselves from other horses or even from people and that come across as very reserved. They are typically loners who, when ill, withdraw into themselves straightaway. They tolerate contact with other horses and familiar people only reluctantly, their body language gives very clear signals of inapproachability and distance. These horses do not come into conflict with other horses as they go out of their way to avoid any proximity. On a physical level, throat and back tension is very common in these horses. Water Violet is often used for horses that have been neglected or stabled alone.

Water Violet, the flower of communication, helps these horses to be able to form relationships and to tolerate closeness. In a positive state, the horses become more sociable and seek out contact with other horses.

Symptoms and uses
- Aggression
- Allergies (to accompany treatment)
- Problems in adjusting
- Arrogance
- Arthritis, arthrosis (to accompany treatment)
- Sensitivity to contact with others
- Aloofness
- Obstinacy
- Propensity for solitude
- Lack of interest
- Isolation
- Problems making contact with other horses
- Strong self-confidence
- Pride
- Inapproachability
- Reserve
- Tension
- Seclusion

Water Violet

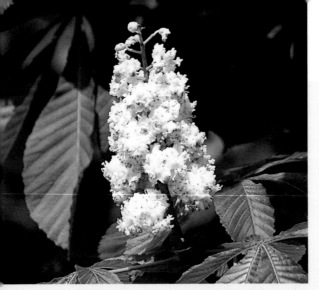

White Chestnut – The flower of reflection. Photo: IPO

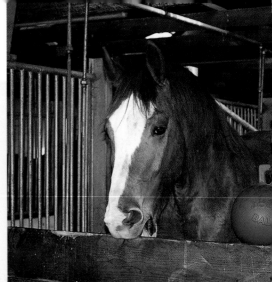

The White Chestnut-horse reveals its great inner tension through behaviour disorders like wind-sucking for example. Photo: Bolze

35. White Chestnut

White Chestnut-horses come across as restless and unbalanced; they appear to be under a great deal of strain. They find it very difficult to concentrate and to learn new things, they are unobservant and appear vacant as well as very tense. If they are ever reprimanded or punished they become despondent very quickly. Often these horses develop stereotypical habits or reveal aggressive behaviour, which is directed towards themselves. Typical symptoms include grinding of teeth, wind-sucking and weaving. White Chestnut is often combined with Vine. The management of the horse should be carefully checked before giving a Bach Flower remedy.

White Chestnut, the flower of reflection, alleviates restlessness and tension; it encourages the horses to concentrate and helps to promote peace. In a positive state, the horses become more balanced, appear calmer within and gain new clarity.

Symptoms and uses

- Distraction
- Strain
- Lethargy
- Illnesses brought about by self aggression
- Periodically recurring illnesses
  (to accompany treatment)
- Exhaustion
- Absentmindedness
- Lack of concentration
- Sensitivity to noise
- Difficulties with learning
- Tiredness
- Despondent character
- Nervousness
- Lack of self-confidence
- Fear of loud noises, sudden bangs
  and bright, flashing lights
- Stubbornness
- Instability
- Susceptibility to accidents
- Restlessness
- Cramps
- Refusal
- Sensitivity to changes in the weather
- Grinding of teeth

White Chestnut

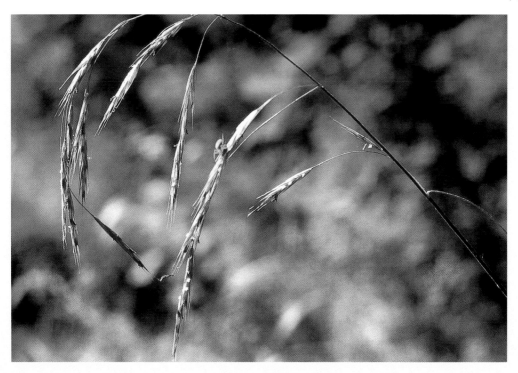

Wild Oat – The flower of purposefulness.
Photo: Institute for Bach Flower Therapy, Andreas Bock

36. Wild Oat

Wild Oat is the appropriate flower for bored and dissatisfied horses who lack stamina. They are often very intelligent and quick to learn new skills. In the short term they can summon up enthusiasm for new things and are very curious, but they quickly lose interest. They find it hard to make friends with other horses since they come across as totally disinterested. During the initial stages of training they co-operate most eagerly but a lack of concentration and indifference soon sets in. They frequently develop forms of substitute behaviour whereby they destroy objects or direct their aggression against themselves. It is important to investigate the management of these horses at the same time as treating them with Bach Flower remedies in order to establish whether this could be contributing to their behaviour. Wild Oat can be

given on its own in cases where several flowers have apparently been necessary or all previous mixtures have not worked.

Wild Oat, the flower of purposefulness, promotes greater stamina and satisfaction. In a positive state, the horses retain their interest in things for much longer. Wild Oat helps to develop more focused behaviour.

Symptoms and uses
- Aggression
- Loss of appetite
- Eye infections (to accompany treatment)
- Lack of stamina
- Short-term ability to be enthusiastic
- Problems with settling in

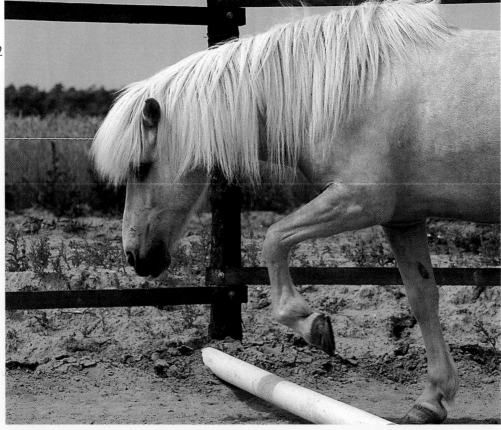

The Wild-Oat horse can show enthusiasm for all new things in the short term but his general disinterest in everything soon reappears.
Photo: Schmelzer

- Propensity for solitude
- Boredom
- Impulsiveness
- Lack of concentration
- Weakness during illness
- Willingness to learn
- Muscular tension (to accompany treatment)
- Nervousness
- Self-destructive behaviour
- Over-enthusiasm
- Inconstency
- Indecision
- Under-stimulated
- Bad habits like wind-sucking or weaving
- Dissatisfaction
- Injuries (to accompany treatment)
- Wounds that fail to heal

37. Wild Rose

Wild Rose is the right flower for listless, apathetic horses that do not show the slightest interest in their lives. They are completely lacking in energy, barely move of their own volition and have a dull expression in their eyes. Their whole appearance reflects their resignation and hopelessness. Motivating them in any way seems impossible. The slightest exertion leads to total exhaustion. The reasons for this often lie in severe illnesses or inappropriate stabling which does not provide these horses with sufficient free room. It is therefore necessary to check how they are managed and give them a thorough physical examination. Wild Rose is also used as an accompanying treatment when dealing with chronic illnesses and it helps to establish whether these horses actually have the will to live.

Wild Rose, the flower of vitality helps create a new joy in life. In a positive state, liveliness is once again restored in these horses; they begin to show an interest in everyday events and are much more easily motivated to become active. Wild Rose promotes a thirst for adventure.

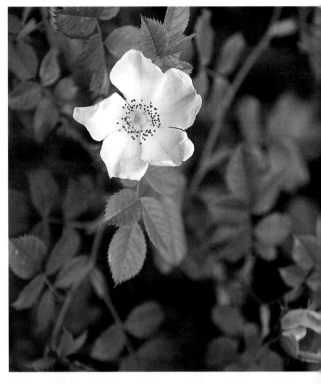

Wild Rose – The flower of vitality. Photo: IPO

Wild Rose helps a resigned, dispirited horse to gain new joy in life.
Photo: Schmelzer

Symptoms and uses

- Weak immune system
- Lack of impetus
- Apathy
- Loss of appetite
- No desire to be active
- Dull expression
- Chronic illnesses (to accompany treatment)
- Disinterest
- Lack of energy
- Exhaustion
- Refusal of food
- Indifference
- Hopelessness
- Susceptibility to illness
- Tiredness
- After a stillbirth
- Unresolved negative experiences
- Weakness
- Euthanasia
- Listlessness
- Injuries (to accompany treatment)
- Tension (to accompany treatment)
- Weakness of will

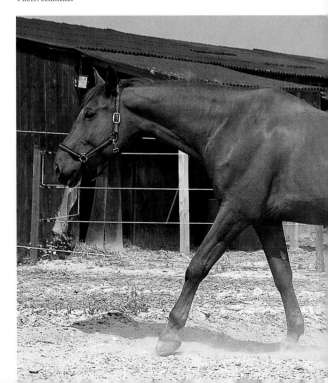

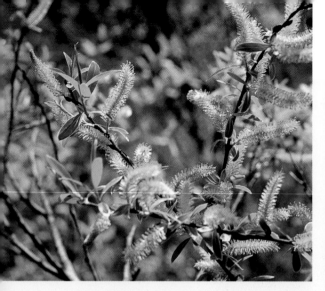

Willow – The flower of fate.
Photo: Institute for Bach Flower Therapy, Andreas Bock

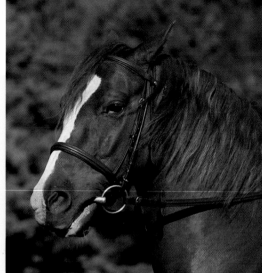

The Willow-horse seems to be permanently bad-tempered and distrustful – mostly due to bad experiences. Photo: Schmelzer

38. Willow

Willow-horses are characterised by their conspicuous bad mood and permanently angry state. It is typical for these horses to keep up a steady, monotonous pawing action. They are very quick to take offence or feel as if they are being attacked and are distrustful, vicious and rebellious. Within the herd these animals are aggressive and hostile. It is quite common to come across these horses that have been mistreated or neglected and, in the vast majority of cases, there needs to be improvements in the way they are managed. Willow is often used in conjunction with Gentian, Holly and Vine.

Willow, the flower of fate, helps these horses to achieve calm and peace. In a positive state, they accept their situation and learn to cope with it better. Willow helps them to relate to people and other horses in a friendlier, more peaceful manner.

Symptoms and uses

- Aggression
- Problems relating to old age
- Quick-tempered disposition
- Rebelliousness
- Biting
- Viciousness
- Problems settling in
- Sensitivity
- Refusal of food
- Anger
- Skin conditions (to accompany treatment)
- Inner restlessness
- Intolerance
- Problems making contact with others
- Moodiness
- Sullenness
- Lack of motivation
- Muscular tension (to accompany treatment)
- Despondent character
- After poor treatment, neglect
- Irritability
- Volatility
- Defiance
- Dissatisfaction
- Bitterness
- Digestion problems
- Rage

39. The special mixture: Rescue Remedy

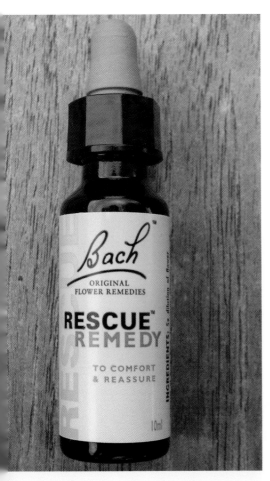

For rapid relief in moments of extreme angst and fear: Rescue Remedy drops. Photo: Bosse

Rescue Remedy drops were conceived for extraordinary situations that have a huge effect on the individual and constitute an emergency for the person involved. They consist of five different flower essences: Cherry Plum for loss of control, Clematis for loss of consciousness, Impatiens for pacifying, Rock Rose for panic and desperation and Star of Bethlehem for shock.

Rescue Remedy drops are not intended to replace veterinary treatment, instead they help to process psychological shock in extreme circumstances. Serious psychological or physical aftereffects can often be prevented by giving Rescue Remedy drops at the right time. They are always advisable when a horse is exposed to a high degree of stress, sudden excitement, threatening situations, or fear and pain – i.e. following an accident, a visit from the farrier or vet, at a competition or even when being ridden by a stranger. It can be applied both internally and externally and the list of conditions it can help with is endless. It is a good idea to always keep the Rescue Remedy close to hand. However, it is important not to use Rescue Remedy for every situation that arises but rather to keep it for emergencies.

The dosage varies depending on the situation in hand: Use five to 10 undiluted drops of Rescue Remedy at a time in short intervals of a few minutes until the animal has become stable. In many cases, a single dose can have an incredibly calming effect.

Rescue Remedy drops are available from chemists as stock bottles in a variety of different sizes.

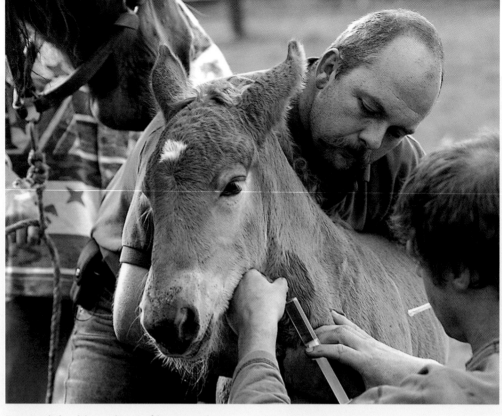

Rescue Remedy drops help to resolve a stressful situation, such as vaccinations, quickly. Photo: Slawik

Rescue Remedy is also available as a spray and a cream, (see page 99) both of which are suitable for external use i.e. for small injuries.

Rescue Remedy drops are often given in emergencies, not only to treat the horse, but also to calm the people involved.

Some examples of usage for Rescue Remedy drops:

- Accidents, injuries
- Before and after operations
- If poisoning is suspected (give Crab Apple first) – until the vet arrives
- Recurring panic attacks
- Fighting within the herd
- Separation from other horses
- Change of stable or owner
- Fear or nervousness before and during transportation
- Competitions
- Mare before being covered
- To help with birth for mares and foals
- Euthanasia (see page 97)
- Cleaning of wounds (externally, mixed with water)
- Removal of ticks (put drops directly onto the ticks or use the spray)

A-Z of problems and suggested treatments

Tip: With tried and tested combinations, the flowers which are to be combined with others have been marked with a '+'.

Abscesses, reddened or covered in pus
- Centaury
- Clematis
- Crab Apple + Olive

Accidents
- Rescue Remedy

Aching muscles
- Elm
- Hornbeam + Olive

Aggression
- Due to a lack of inner stability: Scleranthus
- As a rash reaction: Cherry Plum + Impatiens
- From feelings of jealousy: Holly
- From dominance and an unwillingness to be subordinate: Vine

Allergies
Allergies in animals are often a reaction to a negative environment. It is common to find that horses lacking in self-confidence are not being correctly handled. It is therefore important to investigate and improve the stable management in order to reduce the horse's insecurities.
- Beech
- Rapid and strong allergic reaction: Holly
- Food allergies: Impatiens
- After having been subjected to poor stable management: Mustard
- Raw sensitivity: Crab Apple
- Allergic shock: Rock Rose
- Following a highly traumatic experience: Star of Bethlehem

Allergies, chronic
- Cleansing: Crab Apple, Beech + Holly
- To allow the reaction to be expressed in other ways and to enable the body to alter the current situation: Walnut
- To process the shock which caused the violent reaction: Star of Bethlehem

Allergies, severe
- Initial treatment: Rescue Remedy
- Strong, uncontrollable defensive reactions caused by a rejection of "strangers": Beech
- To aid the removal of harmful substances: Crab Apple

Apathy
- After a frightening situation: Wild Rose
- After a shock: Star of Bethlehem
- Lack of vitality and pleasure in life: Clematis
- Resignation following the loss of another horse or person: Gorse
- Following a serious, physical illness: Olive
- Problems in settling into a new environment: Honeysuckle

Appetite, loss of
- As a means of stimulating and strengthening the horse when excited/agitated: Chicory
- For initial problems with the digestive tract: Crab Apple
- For a general boost: Olive + Walnut

Belligerence
- For aggression: Holly
- For an excessive need to be praised: Vine
- For isolation and obvious inability to make contact with others: Water Violet

- For permanently defeated animals: Sweet Chestnut
- For animals who always want to be the centre of attention: Heather

Birth
- Rescue Remedy
- In preparation for birth: Elm, Chestnut Bud
- After the birth for mares and foals: Star of Bethlehem + Walnut
- After a difficult birth: initially Rock Rose
- After a stillbirth: Rescue Remedy

Choosing the right Bach Flower remedy mixture can be beneficial for both mares and foals as it helps them adjust to their new way of life. Photo: Schomburg

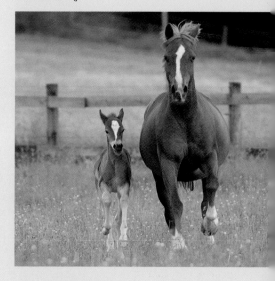

Bronchitis, acute
Consult your vet!
- To accompany treatment: Beech, Olive, Gentian, Hornbeam + Rock Rose

Castration
- Before and after the operation: Rescue Remedy
- Initially: Holly + Honeysuckle + Walnut

Chronic illnesses
- Centaury
- Olive
- Sweet Chestnut
- Vine + Wild Rose

Clumsiness
- Increased when frantic or nervous: Impatiens
- For inertia and lack of motivation: Hornbeam

Colic
- Until the vet arrives: Rescue Remedy every 15 minutes
- Initially: Vervain + Heather
- Frequent colic caused by changes in the weather: Chestnut Bud

Compulsive behaviour
- To encourage tolerance of the prevailing situation: Beech
- To combat excessive behaviour: Impatiens
- To combat addictive tendencies: Chestnut Bud + White Chestnut
- To combat an obstinate, iron will: Oak + Vine
- To promote a receptiveness to new ways of behaving: Walnut + Wild Oat

Concentrating, difficulties with
- Well-known manoeuvres are repeatedly forgotten: Chestnut Bud
- Lack of motivation and interest: Clematis
- Physical and/or mental exhaustion: Hornbeam
- After having survived an illness tiredness: Olive
- Uncertainty and forgetfulness: White Chestnut

Coughing
Essential to consult a vet!
It is advisable to investigate the stable management when dealing with a horse whose cough is caused by an allergy.
- Chestnut Bud + Clematis + Gentian

Cracked hooves
- Mix Tea Tree and Jojoba oil together and combine with Crab Apple, Olive and Walnut. Clean the affected areas and apply the oil mixture thinly.

Cramp
- Rock Water + Chestnut Bud

Depression
- Apparent severe depression: Elm
- Grief caused by loss and problems accepting new things: Walnut
- Sudden, inexplicable loss of pleasure in life: Mustard + Wild Oat
- Despondent behaviour after being reprimanded: Willow
- Lack of self-confidence, depression after being told off: Pine

Destructive mania
- Due to anger or high spirits: Holly (possibly combined with Pine + Willow)
- Excessive nibbling: Impatiens + White Chestnut

Development disorders
- Chestnut Bud
- As a result of yearning for the past: Honeysuckle
- To strengthen the horse's will: Gentian
- As a result of having tried to gain affection by force: Heather

Diabetes

- Processing of inner conflicts: Agrimony
- To increase strength: Olive
- To aid recovery: Gorse

Diarrhoea

- Cherry Plum
- Crab Apple
- Vervain + Scleranthus
- When agitated: Aspen, Impatiens,
  Mimulus + Rock Rose

Distraction

- Agrimony
- Difficulties with learning new skills and
  concentration: Chestnut Bud

Distrust

- Gentian
- Due to fear and aggression:
  Holly, Mimulus and Willow

Eczema

- To get rid of poisonous substances:
  Crab Apple + Chestnut Bud
- To promote healing, especially of skin
  allergies: Wild Rose
- To strengthen the horse's ability to react: Walnut
- To support the body's ability to heal
  itself: Olive

Euthanasia

- To help ascertain whether there is
  still a will to live: Hornbeam, Olive,
  Rescue Remedy + Wild Rose
- To ease the transition and enable the
  animal to be put to sleep peacefully:
  Rescue Remedy, Rock Water + Walnut.

Exhaustion, to aid

See "Recovery"

Fear

- Timid horses who lack confidence: Agrimony
- Animals who are fearful from birth
  onwards: Aspen
- Fear of known things/situations: Mimulus
- Constant fear as a result of bad experiences:
  Sweet Chestnut
- Fear which increases when the animal is
  in shock: Rock Rose
- Fear with hopelessness and a dwindling will
  to live: Wild Rose
- To increase self-confidence and will, to battle
  against fear: Gentian + Larch

Fever

- Rescue Remedy
- Cherry Plum
- Holly + Impatiens

Food envy

- Aggression: Holly
- Due to lack of nutrition in the past:
  Mimulus + Aspen
- To combat inner compulsions: White Chestnut
- To combat a strong, uncontrollable will: Oak
- To combat despair which is displayed as
  jealousy: Cherry Plum

Fungal infections

- To strengthen the immune system: Crab Apple
- To apply externally: use a cleansing mixture
  containing Rescue Remedy + Crab Apple

Heatstroke

- Rescue Remedy

Homesickness
- Base flower: Walnut
- To prevent bitterness developing: Willow
- Lack of acceptance of new surroundings induced by fear: Cherry Plum
- To promote receptiveness to new people and surroundings: Clematis + Cerato
- Overcoming sadness: Honeysuckle
- To ease the settling in process: Hornbeam
- To encourage the horse to get used to changes: Scleranthus

Imbalance
- Agrimony + Cherry Plum

Immune system, strengthening of the
- Centaury, Clematis
- Crab Apple
- Hornbeam
- Larch + Olive

Impatience, irritability, cantankerousness
- Impatiens

In emergencies
- Rescue Remedy

Inertia
- To increase interest: Clematis
- To increase defence mechanisms at the onset of an illness: Rescue Remedy + Crab Apple + Mustard + Olive
- For listless horses: Gorse, Honeysuckle, Pine + Rescue Remedy
- For joy and the ability to make contact with others: Water Violet
- To combat the feeling of self-surrender: Wild Rose
- To combat exhaustion: Olive
- To develop new vitality: Gorse
- To increase self-confidence: Cerato

Infectious diseases
- To aid the healing process at the onset of the infection: Rescue Remedy
- To fight the pathogenic illness: Crab Apple
- To strengthen resistance to illness: Centaury
- To boost strength and optimism: Hornbeam
- Proven mixture: Crab Apple + Holly + Rescue Remedy + Sweet Chestnut

Inflammations
- Oak (also as a compress)

Insect stings, tick bites
- Apply Rescue Remedy to the sting (drops, spray or cream)

Irritability
- Base mixture for problems with aggression and dominance: Holly + Vine
- Due to fear: Aspen + Mimulus
- For difficulties in adjusting on a social level: Water Violet
- For bitterness: Willow
- To regain stability: Impatiens

Jealousy
- As a mixture: Chicory + Heather + Holly + Mimulus + Vine

Jumpiness
- In cases where the horse is repeatedly frightened by familiar things: Mimulus
- To increase the horse's ability to adjust: Beech

Lethargy
- Due to a general lack of interest:
  Clematis + Mustard
- From exhaustion: Hornbeam, Olive

Liver conditions
- To support detoxification: Chicory + Crab Apple

Loneliness, feelings of desolation
- Feelings of constantly being left alone:
  Aspen + Mimulus
- Extreme dependence on owner: Cerato + Heather

Loners
- Horses that lack the ability to make
  contact with others in the herd: Rock Water +
  Water Violet
- Unconscious and inexplicable fears: Aspen
- To increase self-confidence: Larch
- For leaders who dominate: Vervain + Vine

Making contact, difficulties in
- Following a change of stable or problems
  within the herd: Beech

Moodiness
- Dissatisfaction due to over-exertion: Wild Oat
- Strong, short-lived mood swings: Impatiens
- Indecision: Scleranthus
- To strengthen zest for life when dealing with
  inner dissatisfaction: Hornbeam + Willow

Nervousness
- Basic remedy: Impatiens
- Profound, inner fear: Aspen + Mimulus
- Due to rejection of affection: Heather
- Highly sensitive to external influences:
  Crab Apple

- Due to indecision: Scleranthus
- Increased aggression: Holly

Obstinacy
- Distinct stubbornness: White Chestnut
- To promote openness and interest: Clematis
- To bring a sense of balance: Oak
- To help the horse to focus on other living
  things in his surroundings: Vine
- To promote the ability to concentrate:
  Chestnut Bud
- For horses that seem to be in a permanent
  state of high tension and therefore are
  oblivious to their environment: Impatiens

Old age, problems relating to
- Hornbeam
- Oak + Olive + Walnut (eases the transition
  into retirement)

Operations
- Before the operation: Rescue Remedy
- After the operation: Gorse, Hornbeam,
  Mimulus + Olive

Over-sensitivity
- Panic, nervousness and frantic behaviour:
  Rock Rose
- Insecure when left alone: Heather
- To moderate violent reactions: Impatiens
- To improve general stability: Walnut

Pain
- Severe: Rescue Remedy
- To reduce the animal's tendency to become
  increasingly aggressive when in pain: Holly

Panic attacks
- Rescue Remedy

Parasitic infestation
- Crab Apple
- After worming treatment: Centaury
- As a preventative measure: Crab Apple + Walnut

Phantom pregnancy
- Clematis
- Red Chestnut
- Walnut + Wild Oat

Physical strain
- Agrimony

Poisoning
- In serious cases, to activate the body's own healing powers: Rescue Remedy
- Removal of poisonous substances: Crab Apple
- For hopelessness, to increase powers of endurance: Gentian, Sweet Chestnut

Pregnancy
- To help the horse adjust to the new situation: Walnut
- To increase joy in the birth and in the new maternal role: Wild Oat
- To relieve the liver and kidneys: Crab Apple
- For optimism and good humour: Mimulus

Purification/detoxication
- Crab Apple
- Chicory + Clematis

Recovery, to aid
- For general exhaustion: Centaury

- After a long illness: Olive, Oak, Elm, Gorse + Sweet Chestnut
- When the horse retreats because of exhaustion: Hornbeam + Olive
- To increase strength: Olive
- To speed up the removal of poisonous substances: Crab Apple
- To prevent the illness becoming established and to support the healing process: White Chestnut

Restlessness
- Agrimony
- Cherry Plum + Impatiens
- Severe strain (possible grinding of teeth also): White Chestnut

Revitalisation
- After a long illness or having been confined to the stable as the result of an accident: Centaury + Olive

Saddle sores
Let the bruises heal as well as checking whether the saddle fits correctly!
- For external use: Apply a cleansing mixture of Rescue Remedy + Crab Apple

Sadness
- Due to being separated from the herd or at the loss of another horse: Honeysuckle, Larch + Mustard.
- Acute cases: Rescue Remedy

Self-confidence, lack of
- Cerato

Self-destructive behaviour
- Breaking through stereotypical behaviour: Chestnut Bud + White Chestnut
- For self-aggression: Beech + Holly
- To strengthen the will to recover: Rescue Remedy
- For allergies: Crab Apple
- To consolidate mood: Mustard
- For bad habits that are self-destructive, to increase attentiveness: Heather

Self pity
- Heather
- Mimulus + Larch

Sensitivity, excessive
- Aspen

Sensitivity to changes in the weather
- Aspen
- Chestnut Bud
- Scleranthus + Walnut

Sexual disorders
- Mares: Aspen + Pine

Shock
- Rescue Remedy

Stamina, lack of
- Agrimony
- Elm
- Hornbeam
- Olive
- Scleranthus

Stereotypical behaviour
- Due to intense fear: Aspen + Mimulus

- To increase self-confidence: Cerato
- To remind the horse of its innate capabilities: Elm
- To strengthen powers of endurance and increase receptiveness to new experiences: Gentian
- To increase drive and pleasure in new experiences: Wild Rose
- To develop decisiveness: Scleranthus
- In acute cases: Rescue Remedy

Stress
- Base flower: Cherry Plum
- Due to fear of a threat: Rescue Remedy

Submissiveness
- Centaury

Summer eczema (sweet itch)
- Crab Apple
- Olive
- Walnut + Wild Rose

A horse suffering from sweet itch will rub against every available object to try and ease the excruciating itching. Photo: van Damsen

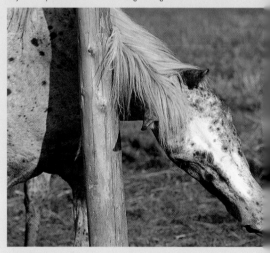

Sunstroke
- Rescue Remedy

Tension
- To promote the ability to "let go":
  Cherry Plum + Oak + Rock Water + Vervain

Transportation
- Rescue Remedy

Not every horse views the prospect of being transported calmly. Rescue Remedy drops can help to diffuse the harrowing situation. Photo: Bosse

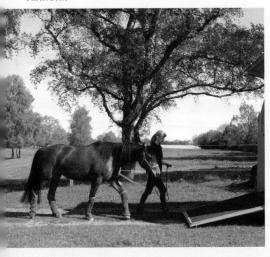

Tumours, growths
- Benign growths: Cerato
- For blocked vitality which is manifested in growths: Agrimony
- To restore the growth to its original function: Wild Oat
- For optimism and acceptance of the condition: Hornbeam
- For the horse who treats his own body with indifference: Clematis

- As a long-term therapy to accompany treatment: Rescue Remedy + Crab Apple + Elm + Olive (Please note: As an exception, Rescue Remedy is used here as a component part of the mixture for long-term use)

Uncertainty
- Cerato + Larch

Viciousness
- Dominant behaviour within the herd or towards people: Vervain + Vine
- Intolerant animals that seek to impose their will: Beech
- Sudden bouts of aggression and desire to fight: Holly
- Horses that chase away all those who come near them: Water Violet

Weak immune system
- To build up the immune system: Agrimony
- Removal of poisonous substances: Crab Apple
- General strengthening: Centaury, Chicory, Clematis, Larch + Olive

Weakness of will
- Centaury

Willingness to learn, to encourage a
- Chestnut Bud
- Centaury
- Hornbeam + White Chestnut

Wind-sucking
- Cherry Plum
- Chestnut Bud
- Clematis
- Impatiens + White Chestnut

Wounds

- To aid the healing of a wound: Gorse
- General strengthening of the immune system: Hornbeam + Olive
- For gaping, open wounds: Agrimony
- To cleanse wounds: Crab Apple
- For restlessness and impatience: Impatiens
- For situations where the horse disregards his injuries and slows down the healing process: Oak
- When the horse seems to enjoy his special status: Water Violet
- To activate the body's own healing powers: Scleranthus
- If the horse's condition deteriorates suddenly: Sweet Chestnut
- To promote a readiness to accept long-term limitations: Willow

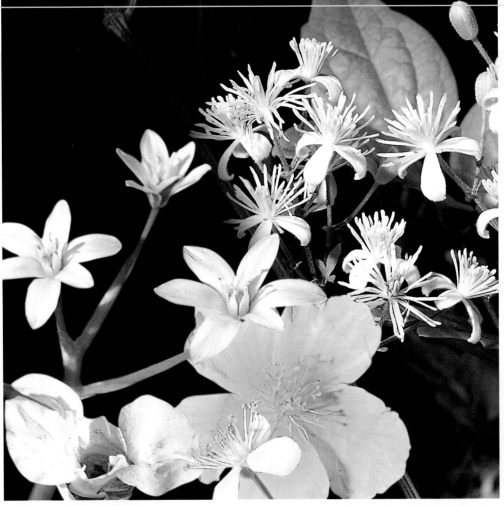

The Rescue Remedy mixture contains the following Bach Flowers: Cherry Plum, Clematis, Impatiens, Rock Rose and Star of Bethlehem.
Photo: Bosse

Proven Bach Flower remedies and mixtures for common problems

Fear

A small incident such as a sudden noise in the riding arena is all it takes to cause a sensitive horse to continue to shy away from a particular area in the future. A single, fleeting moment of fear when being loaded into a horsebox can create permanent problems with transportation for an inexperienced horse. Whatever the cause of the problem, the owner has to regain the horse's trust, in order to resolve the situation. This is true for all cases, whether the owner is dealing with a horse that shies away from water or from saddles, that is frightened of certain obstacles or is just generally apprehensive. This process requires a great deal of patience. You should never expect more from a horse than you are prepared to give. A great many fears arise during training, in situations wherein excessive demands are placed on the horse. The fears generated in this way can only be alleviated if all subsequent contact with the horse is made in an extremely calm manner.

As a preventative measure to deal with severe cases of fear e.g. while the horse is being ridden or during a competition, 8-10 Rescue Remedy drops have proved to be excellent. When the horse is actually taking part in a competition, this should be replaced by either diluted drops or globules (see page 18). A mixture made up of the following flowers is recommended for horses that are permanently shy and fearful:

- **Aspen** – to combat general apprehension and inexplicable fears
- **Cerato** – to combat uncertainty and to increase self-confidence
- **Cherry Plum** – to combat inner tension and restlessness
- **Larch** – to combat lack of courage and despair, to increase self-assurance
- **Mimulus** – as a base flower to combat fear of known things
- **Star of Bethlehem** – to deal with shock

Aggression

Aggressive behaviour towards people is almost always caused by the fact that the horse has been mistreated, poorly managed or simply as a result of excessive demands being placed upon him. In order to treat a horse successfully in the long term it is essential to establish the cause of his behaviour and then improve the situation. These investigations can prove to be futile if a horse has already had several previous owners. In these cases the owner needs to take a step backwards in his approach to the horse and his training and try to regain the horse's trust using calmness and understanding. A rider who treats his horse with compassion and learns to decipher his body language, gives him clear guidelines. This provides him with the security that is so crucial to a horse and it is this security that enables him to accept his owner as the leader of the herd. The following Bach Flowers are recommended to support this process:

- **Beech** – to increase tolerance and combat aggression
- **Cherry Plum** – to combat inner tension and restlessness
- **Star of Bethlehem** – to deal with physical and psychological shock
- **Vine** – to promote compliance within the horse, to combat excessive dominance

If horses are not properly managed, they are unable to form relationships amongst themselves. They then begin to behave in an aggressive and dominant manner towards other horses, may ignore them completely or are indiscriminately friendly. A horse that is kept in a stable all year long consequently interacts with the herd in a disturbed manner; he approaches other horses with either fear or aggression. In order to ease the horse's ability to understand the natural hierarchy of the herd and to offer support in situations arising through power struggles and jealousy, it is initially helpful to add the flower Holly to the above mixture.

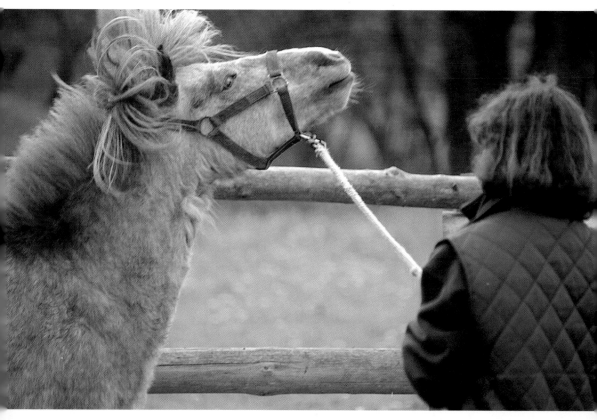

If a horse disobeys a command, the first thing to establish is whether it is due to fear, impatience, obstructiveness or physical pain.
Photo: Schmelzer

Obstructiveness

One of the most common problems arising in the relationship between man and horse is when the horse is obstructive, either when being ridden or on a day-to-day basis.

Eight to ten drops of Rescue Remedy can be given in severe cases, for example, when a horse is napping from stress, fear or agitation or during a visit from the vet or farrier. In situations where it is possible to foresee problems in advance, the drops should be given a few hours before the event and then repeated on an hourly basis. In certain cases of need, i.e. when the vet is carrying out an unpleasant or painful exami-

nation, the Rescue Remedy drops can be given at short intervals of 15 minutes.

If the horse is refusing to co-operate while being ridden, it is important to rule out the possibility of the horse being in pain. This could be caused either by an ill-fitting saddle or even by the position of the rider. Tension in the back, throat or jaw can often provoke a sudden outburst from the horse or result in an increasing tendency to nap. If everything is as it should be, the Bach Flower remedy should be given as a long-term treatment over several weeks. If you are dealing with a very nervous horse who always reacts to a certain situation by shying away, bucking or attempting to escape because of his inner panic and uncertainty, then a mixture for dealing with fear made up of the following flowers is to be recommended:

- **Aspen** – to combat general jumpiness and inexplicable fears
- **Cerato** – to increase inner security and self-confidence
- **Gentian** – to combat fear and distrust of new and unknown things
- **Larch** – to increase self-assurance and the horse's faith in his own abilities
- **Mimulus** – to combat specific fears and fear of known things and situations
- **Star of Bethlehem** – to deal with the possibility of negative experiences in the past

If the horse's tendency to nap is not caused by fear but instead lies in his need to dominate, the following Bach Flower mixture has proved helpful. It is effective for horses that are inclined to battle with their rider and refuse to co-operate:

- **Beech** – to combat aggression, intolerance and an excessive will, to reduce the desire to fight and propensity for protesting
- **Cherry Plum** – for sudden temperamental outbursts and volatility
- **Holly** – to combat rage, hostility and aggression
- **Vervain** – to combat inner nervousness, impulsiveness and restlessness
- **Vine** – reduces dominance, obstinacy and tyrannical behaviour

If the horse appears frantic, impatient and easily irritated it is advisable to add **Impatiens.**

Bad habits and compulsive behaviour

The best-known and most prevalent displays of compulsive behaviour are wind sucking and weaving. Wind-sucking is a sign of disturbed behaviour that occurs as a result of boredom and loneliness. In some cases it is also viewed as a substitute for foals whose suckling period was too short or did not happen at all. Wind-sucking horses wear down their incisors in an uneven fashion. They are often finicky eaters and regularly suffer from problems linked to the digestive tract (such as colic), which means that the vet needs to be called out on a regular basis. Common methods for dealing with the problem such as using a strap, tethering the horse, hanging up sandbags or even deciding to have the horse operated on, merely suppress the symptoms of the disorder. In order to actually resolve the problem these methods must go hand-in-hand with distinct changes in the way the horse is managed. It is important to look at ways of creating more movement or variety, which seems to encourage the horse to refrain from indulging in these forms of stereotypical behaviour and also help him to cope with his situation. It is best to try and deal with the problems in the initial stages before it becomes a habit.

A weaving horse often spends hours moving his head from side to side and constantly shifting from one foreleg to the other. This can cause permanent damage to the legs and more importantly, can have a damaging effect on the horse's soul.

Another common problem with horses is their tendency to gnaw wood. It is important to check whether their diet may be lacking in raw food or mineral salts and to rectify this if necessary.

Gnawing is frequently caused by a lack of stimulus for the horse, insufficient contact with other horses or constant exposure to stressful situations. In these circumstances, a horse's tendency to gnaw on wood whenever possible is perceived as a form of disturbed behaviour and the first course of action to treat this must be to improve the management of the horse. Access to non-toxic woody plants while grazing or in the stable can contribute to satisfying the horse's instinct for play.

The following Bach Flower mixture can be helpful, in addition to the measures mentioned above, to treat these forms of compulsive behaviour:

- **Cherry Plum** – to combat inner tension
- **Chestnut Bud** – to combat restlessness and to help to put an end to unreasonable behaviour.
- **Clematis** – promotes an awareness of everyday life
- **Impatiens** – to combat impatience and inner turbulence
- **Vine** – to combat inner aggression and compulsions
- **White Chestnut** – to combat compulsive behaviour

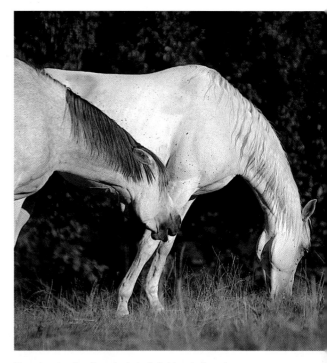

Every time there is a change in the herd, the hierarchy has to be readjusted. Photo: Schmelzer

Problems within the herd

Horses are herd animals and in a group they create a distinct hierarchy in competitive situation, such as around feeding areas, popular resting places, or when they come to drink, which is clearly visible to the trained eye. Harmony does not always reign within a community out in the field. The pecking order is disturbed with each new arrival and the new horse has to find his place within the herd. By initially separating new horses from the rest of the herd with a fence, they can get to know each other in a non-threatening manner. This also serves to reduce the possibilities of any psychological confrontation developing. Problems are often caused if a horse takes a long time to settle into the herd. Domineering leaders (Vervain or Vine-horses) frequently tyrannise unsure and weaker horses.

To support a fearful horse that is lacking in self-confidence, the following mixture can be given:

- **Aspen** – to combat inexplicable fears
- **Gentian** – to combat wariness of all new things
- **Larch** – to increase self-confidence
- **Mimulus** – to combat fear of new things
- **Star of Bethlehem** – to be able to resolve negative experiences from the past

Pine is also recommended for horses that are very submissive, are constantly subordinated and give the impression of being very guilty.

The following mixture has been successful in helping herd leaders that are too aggressive and domineering to achieve greater tolerance and pliability:

- **Beech** – to reduce excessive will, arrogance and aggressive tendencies
- **Cherry Plum** – to combat inner tension
- **Holly** – to promote tolerance
- **Impatiens** – to combat impatience and irritability
- **Vervain** – to reduce excessive behaviour and impulsiveness
- **Vine** – to combat aggression, dominance and tyrannical behaviour

To aid the healing process in injuries and illnesses

Bach Flower remedies can be used to aid the healing process in every type of illness and injury. However, they are not intended to replace treatment by a vet! The following mixtures are proven remedies:

Allergies, all types of skin complaints and infestations by parasites

- **Rescue Remedy** – the first thing to be taken for severe outbreaks of allergies
- **Beech** – base flower for allergies, to combat severe rashes
- **Crab Apple** – to promote detoxification and the release of toxins

- **Holly** – for the sudden appearance of severe cases of allergies
- **Impatiens** – for food allergies
- **Rock Rose** – for allergic shocks
- **Walnut** – to help a horse deal with a new situation

Applying the Bach Flower remedies externally can also be effective when dealing with eczema, rashes and all superficial skin conditions.

Severe or chronic respiratory illnesses

- **Beech** – base flower for allergies
- **Centaury** – to promote the will to recover
- **Hornbeam** – to increase strength and energy
- **Olive** – to combat inner exhaustion

Diarrhoea and constipation

- **Olive** – to increase strength and energy
- **Scleranthus** – alternating diarrhoea and constipation
- **Vervain** – to combat inner nervousness

Colic and poisoning

- **Rescue Remedy** – the first thing to give while waiting for the vet to arrive
- **Crab Apple** – to remove poisonous substances
- **Gentian** – to strengthen powers of endurance
- **Olive** – to increase strength
- **Sweet Chestnut** – to increase the will to recover

Wounds and injuries

- **Rescue Remedy** – first thing to give
- **Crab Apple** – as a form of cleansing
- **Gorse** – to aid the healing of wounds
- **Hornbeam** – to strengthen the immune system
- **Impatiens** – to combat inner restlessness
- **Olive** – to increase strength and energy

All types of infectious illnesses

- **Rescue Remedy** – to give support at the onset of the infection
- **Centaury** – to promote resistance
- **Crab Apple** – to fight pathogens, to help release toxins
- **Hornbeam** – to provide vitality, strength and optimism

To promote vitality and a zest for life

The following Bach Flower mixtures are recommended for veteran horses or for horses that are either suffering from a long illness or convalescing. They serve to provide new strength and energy and to restore vitality:

- **Clematis** – to activate pleasure in life
- **Crab Apple** – to strengthen the immune system
- **Elm** – to combat exhaustion and despondency
- **Gorse** – to increase strength and motivate the horse to persevere
- **Honeysuckle** – to fight sadness and apathy
- **Hornbeam** – brings new energy, to combat tiredness
- **Olive** – to strengthen vitality and provide energy

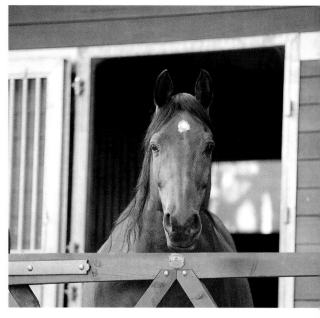

A change of stable or owner can be a traumatic experience for a horse. Bach Flower remedies help the horse to accept the new situation. Photo: van Damsen

Homesickness following a change of stable or owner

The first traumatic event experienced by the horse is usually being weaned and then separated from his mother; in many cases this separation also involves a change of yard or owner. The foal requires a great deal of love and patience during this phase in order to come to trust his new owner, as he has to make enormous adjustments.

A change of stable or owner, which involves being separated from other familiar horses, can also be highly traumatic even for fully-grown horses. The sadness that is linked to this experience can often result in apathetic or aggressive behaviour.

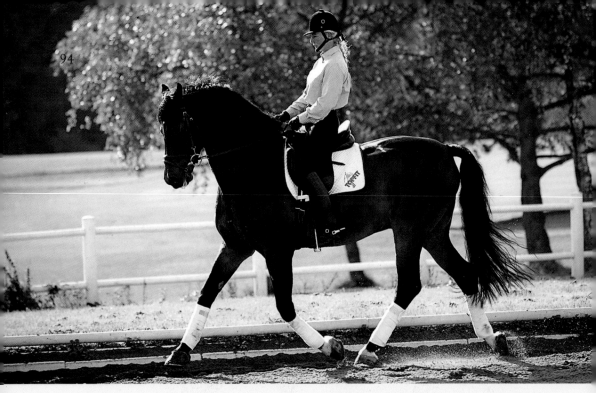

A rider can only demand and expect full co-operation from the horse if his level of training and strength have been taken into account in his schooling programme. Photo: Prohn

Difficulties with learning and training

The following Bach Flower mixture helps the horse to let go of the past more easily, work through the separation and adjust to his new life:

- **Honeysuckle** – helps with new beginnings
- **Star of Bethlehem** – to deal with shock
- **Walnut** – to combat insecurity
  in the new situation

The following can be added to the mixture as necessary:

- **Aspen and Mimulus** – for sudden fear
  and uncertainty
- **Water Violet** – for difficulties in adjusting
  to the new herd

When looking for a Bach Flower remedy for difficulties with learning new skills, it is important to rule out the possibility of excessive demands being placed upon the horse. If the rider is extremely ambitious and the programme does not cater for the horse's age, level of training and ability, the horse can suffer from what is known as 'burnout syndrome', which in turn leads to tiredness, lethargy and even to a downright refusal to co-operate. However, if the expectations are reasonable, the horse is being trained by an experienced rider and is still distracted, forgetful and derives no pleasure at all from the work, then the following mixture may help:

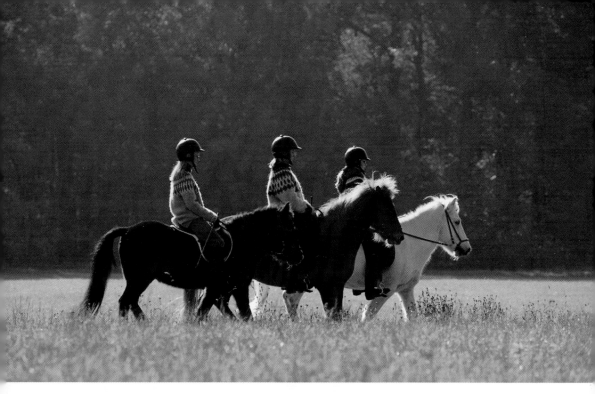

A ride should be like this – a balm for people and for the horse's soul. Photo: van Damsen

- **Agrimony** – to combat distraction and to encourage concentration
- **Centaury** – for lack of concentration and sudden tiredness
- **Chestnut Bud** – for clumsiness and carelessness, to foster awareness
- **Hornbeam** – to combat tiredness and lethargy, help with motivation and energy, especially for horses who switch off in routine lessons but who are eager to co-operate when learning something new
- **White Chestnut** – to promote concentration and a willingness to learn, to combat tiredness and absent-mindedness
- **Wild Oat** – to combat moodiness, when the horse loses interest very quickly

Problems when being ridden

Dealing with rearing, bucking, lashing out, constant shying away or bolting while out hacking in the countryside is not only tiresome and unpleasant, but also dangerous for man and horse alike.

It is crucial to distinguish between bad habits which occur because of fear or insecurity as opposed to arising from disobedience, anger or aggression. As the rider's own insecurity (in anticipating problems) often plays a huge part in the situation, they too should take a suitable Bach Flower mixture. It goes without saying that only highly experienced and competent riders should go out hacking on such unpredictable horses. On a similar note it is crucial to ensure that the horse receives a thorough training in the indoor school and in the arena. The bad habits that many horses display while hacking also emerge while they are

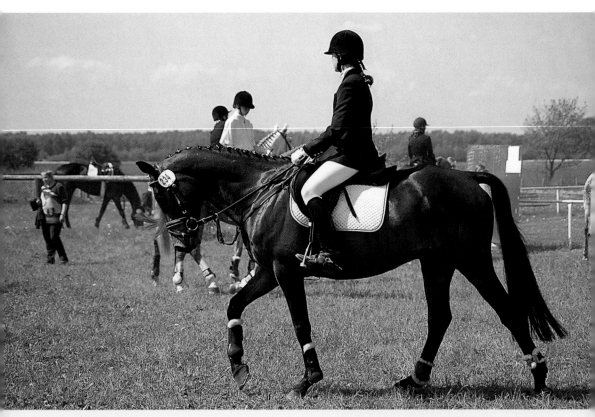

Competitions are often highly stressful for both the horse and rider. The right Bach Flower remedy helps turn nerves into stability. Photo:Wedekind

working and should be addressed in training.

The following is recommended to temper the situation:

- **Rescue Remedy** – (eight to 10 drops) before or during the ride as necessary

It is also advisable to give the following Bach Flower mixture over a long period of time, depending on the horse's temperament:

- **Aspen, Cherry Plum, Gentian, Mimulus, Rock Rose** – for nervous horses
- **Beech, Holly, Vervain, Vine** – for aggressive and dominant horses

Heather can also be added if the horse has a tendency to stick to other horses while hacking.

Competitions

Many horses are enthusiastic and willing to learn in their daily training sessions and cause no problems at all when being handled. However, as soon as preparations begin on the day of the competition, they suffer from a great deal of inner tension, which is expressed in nervous or anxious behaviour. Horses are very perceptive and can pick up on the rider's excitement before a competition. Therefore it is important to ensure that all preparations are carried out calmly at a measured pace to avoid unsettling highly sensitive horses. The owner should make sure that the horse has practiced loading into the horsebox plenty of times in advance and also that enough time has been allotted for this. It is better to avoid recruiting lots of well-meaning helpers to assist at this stage. In most cases it is advisable for the rider and, if need be, other people involved with the event to take a suitable Bach Flower mixture in order to remain calm.

Rescue Remedy drops should be given to both horse and rider at the first acute signs of stress or nervousness. It is a good idea to use Rescue Remedy globules for the horse before and during the competition (see page 18).

In addition to this, particularly agitated or nervous horses would benefit from being given the following flowers a long time in advance:
- **Aspen** – for inexplicable fears
- **Mimulus** – for fear of known things and situations

If the horse has a tendency to be difficult because of a need to dominate, it is also useful to give him these flowers well in advance:
- **Beech** – to combat aggression and protests
- **Holly** – to encourage tolerance, to combat aggression and viciousness
- **Vine** – to combat obstinacy and excessive dominance

Euthanasia and helping the aged horse

Bach Flowers can never kill! They are a very safe and effective means of helping an old or sick horse to come to his own decision as to whether he wants to keep living or pass away. They also reduce fear and can ease the transition.

A horse that appears withdrawn and apathetic, refuses food and water and seems to be lacking in motivation, can be given a combination of Rescue Remedy drops, Hornbeam, Wild Rose and Olive to establish whether he still has the will to live. If there is a change within the next 30 minutes, if the horse becomes motivated again and reacts to someone talking to him, possible by wiggling his ears, then, on a spiritual level, he may not yet have made the decision to leave this life. It is definitely worth trying to revive him with conventional medicine.

If the horse continues to behave in an apathetic manner despite having been given the Bach Flower remedy, it is then possible to ease his situation with a mixture of Rescue Remedy drops, Walnut and Rock Water. In this way you may make it possible for him to pass away peacefully, in familiar surroundings. The horse will decide himself when that time is to be.

The same mixture can be used if the vet is called to put the animal to sleep. It ensures that the horse's psyche is at peace before the sedative is given and thus plays an important part in making sure that the animal is physically calm. The Bach Flower remedy serves to comfort such animals and they radiate an extraordinary aura of peace in their last moments.

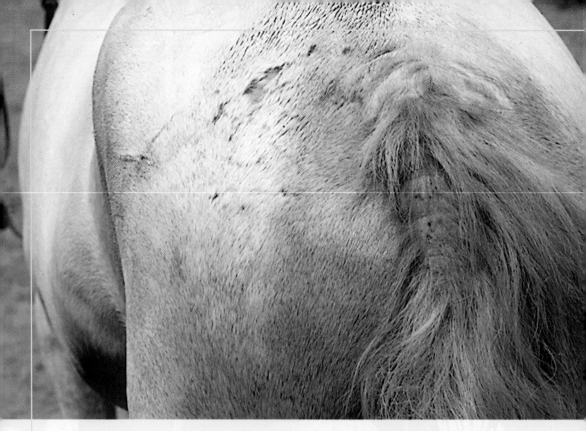

Bach Flower remedies have also proved effective for dealing with sweet itch, when applied externally.
Photo: Clinic for working animals, Bern

External application of Bach Flower remedies

Compresses, cleansing tonics and poultices

In addition to being taken internally, Bach Flowers can also be used as cold compresses and poultices. For these external uses add six drops of the appropriate flowers to 500ml of still water.

Recommendation:

• To wean foals: Crab Apple, Walnut (spray or cleanse the teats with the mixture as well as giving mares and foals the remedy internally)

- Skin complaints, eczema: Beech, Crab Apple
- Inflammations, also on joints:
  Beech, Crab Apple, Oak
- Injuries: (bruises, contusions, sprains,
  pulled ligaments or muscles):
  Rescue Remedy, Crab Apple
- Insect bites: Rescue Remedy
- Sweet itch: Beech, Crab Apple, Hornbeam

To create a tonic to protect against insect bites, use a mixture of water and vinegar (three litres of water to one litre of vinegar) and add six drops of Crab Apple and Centaury respectively.

Hot compresses with Crab Apple, Oak, Rescue Remedy and Rock Water are effective for circulatory problems as well as releasing tension in problems with muscles and joints.

Eye drops made from boiled water and Crab Apple (four drops in 20ml water and allowed to cool) have proven helpful in dealing with conjunctivitis.

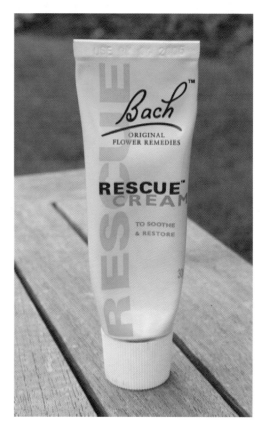

Photo: Bosse

Rescue cream

Bach Flower Rescue cream is available from chemists and is lanolin free and unperfumed. In addition to the Rescue Remedy flowers Clematis, Cherry Plum, Impatiens, Rock Rose and Star of Bethlehem, it also contains the flower Crab Apple (the cleansing flower).

Rescue cream can be used for a wide variety of injuries. It helps to speed up the healing process if applied to cuts and grazes. When dealing with open wounds, it should only be applied to the edge of the wound. This cream is also worth a try for skin conditions, insect bites and all kinds of eczema. If used swiftly in acute cases, it works as an analgesic and reduces swelling and infections.

To produce your own Rescue cream, mix two drops of Rescue Remedy and a drop of Crab Apple in 10ml of a neutral ointment (available from the chemist). If you need to reduce swelling, add Holly.

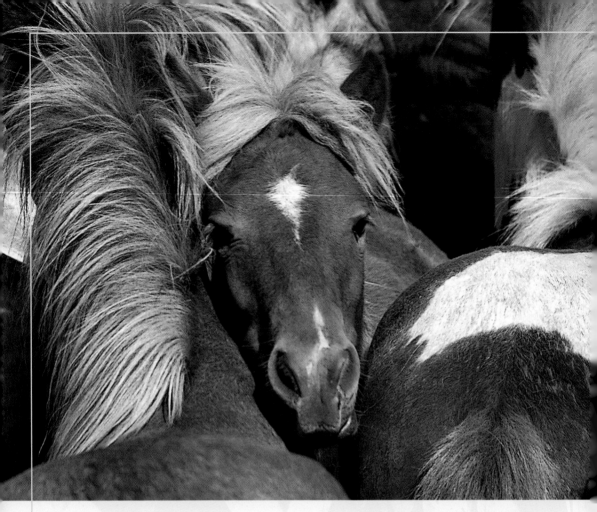

As a herd animal, the horse needs to be in contact with other horses for his psychological well-being. Photo: Schmelzer

Fundamental conditions for successfully treating horses with Bach Flowers

The vast majority of all bad habits and behavioural disorders are avoidable. They arise when the horse's fundamental needs as a herd animal that is instinctively poised for flight are not being met. This can either be in terms of the way they are managed or in their training and the people who are dealing with the horse are, therefore, ultimately responsible.

It is impossible to compensate for poor management or mistreatment by using Bach Flower remedies. In order to alleviate physical or psychological damage that has been caused by inadequate management, then the external factors must be improved first. It is only once all these changes have been effected that Bach Flower remedies can be given. They allow the horse to work through the negative experiences he has had in the past and help to restore psychological balance.

Every responsible horse owner should therefore endeavour to provide his horse with a way of life that is completely in keeping with his needs. This is essential whatever his own ambitions for the horse may be. One of the horse's most pressing requirements is to be able to spend time out in the field with other horses.

The horse's instincts and psyche

A balanced psyche is crucial for the horse's well-being, health, capability and performance. Each horse is an individual, is either sensitive or robust, and has developed specific means of overcoming and working through difficulties. Man's job is to understand his horse in order to be able to deal with him appropriately.

Modern horsemanship takes very little notice of the fundamental psychological disposition of the horse as a herd animal that is instinctively poised for flight. Horses are often handled in a way that fails to nurture their instincts and that consequently leads to bad habits or behavioural disorders. Being kept in a stable for long periods of time, frequent changes in the herd and irregular feeding patterns are just a few examples.

Horses that are lethargic, obstinate, lifeless or even vicious when being ridden have often been treated in a manner which taints their behaviour. In the course of their lives, they have been exposed at least once to inadequate or even brutal treatment.

There are different temperaments within the species and it is common to come across volatile, impatient or even stubborn types. However, a horse is rarely born with a psychological disorder. Bad habits have almost always been caused by people – even though it may have been done subconsciously. When the herd fails to provide protection in difficult situations, and the horse cannot relate to the rider, the horse's psyche seeks an outlet for its stress or fear. Every single display of disturbed behaviour such as wind-sucking, weaving, shying away, or rearing is a cry for help.

If the owner is aware of the reasons for the horse's behaviour and amends the way the horse is managed, almost all these bad habits will be corrected in the process. Since horses develop friendships and conflicts arise between them in the herd, it is often helpful to change the size and composition of the group when feuds occur.

Social structures should also be taken into consideration when organising stabling. Two horses that clash out in the field should not be put in neighbouring stables. Similarly, horses that have become friends should be placed as close to one another as possible.

In order to enable the rider to separate his horse from the group, and to be able to go out riding alone on occasions, it is important for the horse to get used to being separated from the herd regularly as early as possible. This goes against deep-rooted herd instincts. As soon as the horse is weaned he can learn that when he is separated from his mother for short intervals, he always sees her again. If he is then isolated from the herd on a regular basis, he will gradually come to accept the situation. A horse that is schooled in this manner does not lose his instinct but instead develops a firm trust in his owner.

It is then possible to ride without being accompanied by another horse and, after appropriate training, to go for rides away from the group in the pasture.

Causes and prevention of behavioural disorders

Phlegmatic, stubborn or lazy horses react to stimuli differently than temperamental, nervous or enthusiastic horses. A rider who is unable to draw out the positive, innate tendencies of the horse and reinforces negative behaviour instead, contributes to the development of bad habits. A sensitive horse will become even more nervous when being ridden by an insecure rider and a lazy horse will become even more stubborn and dead to the leg with a weak rider.

A spontaneous reaction from a horse can become a fixed response if the situation is repeated. It you are dealing with a horse whose rider falls off when he bucks, the horse may well repeat this behaviour at the next available opportunity and, if he succeeds a second time, this can lead to behaviour disorders. A 'genuine' form of disturbed behaviour is deemed to exist in situations wherein a horse is exhibiting patterns of behaviour which permanently deviate from the norm, and causes such as pain, fear or problems linked to the hierarchy of the herd have been ruled out. In all other cases, the horse's behaviour is merely a reaction to the fact that his fundamental needs have been disregarded and it is up to the people involved with the horse to intervene on a regular basis.

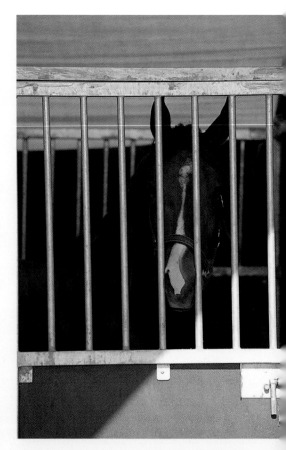

Keeping a horse in a single stable where the windows have bars goes against his instinctive needs. Photo: van Damsen

Behavioural disorders often arise as a result of traumatic experiences. This is frequently referred to as an initial trauma. The social development of the horse can be hampered, for instance, by situations in which the foal is stabled with the mother only and not with other horses. Further causes for the emergence of disturbed behaviour in young horses can be:
- Being weaned too early or too suddenly from the mother
- Beginning training too abruptly
- Being overtaxed during training either on a psychological or spiritual level

- Enforced stable rest due to illness, linked with social isolation
- A change of yard (especially when a young horse, that has been raised in accordance with its needs, is suddenly put into a training yard or a single stable with no familiar horses nearby, or the freedom to move around extensively)

Many horses are exposed to at least one such initial trauma during their lives. Therefore, Star of Bethlehem should be included in almost every mixture for horses. However, not all animals react by developing behaviour disorders. Scientific studies have proved that so-called predisposed factors are jointly responsible for the emergence of disturbed behaviour. Therefore, stable management, daily contact with the horse and genetic influences all have their role to play.

One extremely important factor is the connection with the intense fear that the horse experiences in strange and frightening situations. This fear is based on the horse's instinct to flee at the slightest hint of danger. This is at the root of many of the problems linked to loading a horse onto a horsebox. Young horses are often not given enough time to explore the ramp and dark trailer properly, both of which are potentially frightening for a horse. It is not surprising that the horse, an animal that originally roamed freely, is reluctant to go into the unfamiliar 'black hole' which offers no possibility for flight – in this case a transporter. An initial impulse to bolt or shy away is a normal reaction in a horse and would once have been necessary to ensure its survival. For a horse, losing his balance on uneven ground (i.e. in stretches of water or puddles) or being vulnerable to attack are elements which are linked to this primeval fear. If the horse is not allowed to investigate the situation fully and ascertain that there is no danger, the instinct to flee is increased. Every time he is reprimanded for a reaction prompted by fear, the fear simply increases and this paves the way for severe behavioural disorders. It is important to devote a great deal of time to working with the horse in a highly concentrated manner so that the horse has so much trust in the person that he will allow himself to be guided by them even though it goes against all his instincts.

One point that deserves a mention in avoiding behavioural disorders is that of preventative measures such as selective breeding. Some types of behavioural disorders like wind-sucking, excessive fear or aggression are evident in certain breeds. It is extremely difficult to treat a horse that has inherited patterns of disturbed behaviour and a great deal of emphasis is placed on responsible breeding. Stallions and mares exhibiting disturbed behaviour should consequently be excluded from the breeding programmes if there is evidence that related animals are showing signs of behaviour which deviates from the norm.

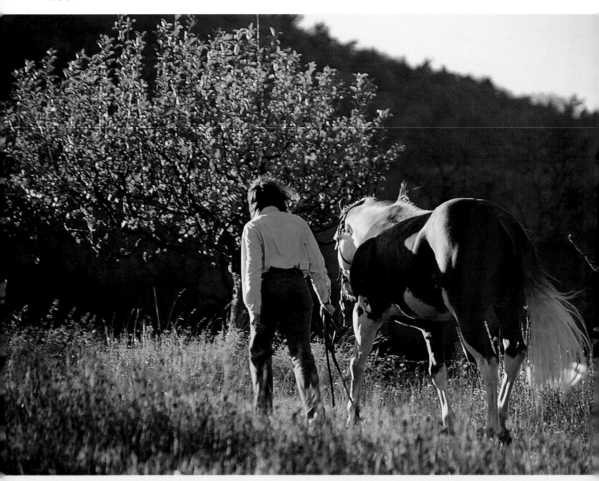

The ideal relationship between man and horse is one of trust and harmony with a clear hierarchy. Photo: Schmelzer

Communication between man and horse

When a horse is being ridden the rider uses his weight, thighs and reins as a method to convey his needs. However, man and horse communicate in a variety of different ways over the course of their daily interaction while the horse is being fed, groomed and managed. If used responsibly, leading reins and whips can be useful when training the horse but there should never be the slightest hint of anger, aggression or violence. Horses are highly sensitive beings: they react swiftly and surely to clear signals from people; they react equally swiftly to major shortcomings in the way they are managed. The psychological distress, which arises as a result of mistreatment, often manifests itself in the form of disturbed behaviour, indefinable fears or aggression.

One of the most important aspects in the relationship between man and horse is the creation of trust – which should be present when out riding as well as in the day-to-day contact on the yard. It is important to train the horse using a series of small steps. This ensures that the horse can successfully master each step and can be warmly praised at every stage.

In order for the horse to feel secure and protected in threatening situations, the person caring for him must hold a position of higher rank. He needs to have a great capacity for understanding and specialised subject knowledge. He also needs to be highly experienced and both firm and consistent in his daily dealings with the horse. It is fundamentally wrong to beat a horse because it does not encourage them to be submissive; it only leads to fear or aggression. If the hierarchy is established at a very early stage and done so in a way which instils a sense of trust in the horse, then he will accept his position and behave accordingly.

To avoid overtaxing the horse, it is important to realise that these animals can only concentrate for a certain length of time. The actual length varies with each horse and depends on their age, level of development, character and the nature of the exercise. Experience shows that young horses can concentrate for a maximum of 10 minutes, and grown animals for up to 20 minutes at a time. The horse will be overburdened if required to work for a whole hour without any breaks. A training programme that fully caters for the animal's needs will take into account each horse's ability to concentrate. Regular breaks on a long rein should be incorporated into every riding hour.

Competition horses out in the field – is this a contradiction?

Some horse owners still believe that, apart from their daily training session, competition horses should remain in their stables, be fed with high-energy food and warmly covered in winter. They should only be turned out into the field when the weather is good and for up to a maximum of one or two hours daily. To avoid possible injuries many people recommend separating them from other horses. The fact that the vet is frequently called out to treat these horses for illnesses such as colic, coughing, and lameness seems, to many of these people, to be purely co-incidental and in explicable.

The truth is that these views go against all the conditions required by the horse to lead a fulfilling life. In view of the fact that its elementary needs are being disregarded, it is hardly surprising that horses managed in this way suffer from frequent illnesses. They are also unfocused when being ridden and express their frustration and their need to be active by refusing to co-operate at competitions.

Each horse has a pressing need for daily exercise, daylight and fresh air, irrespective of his breed and whether he is used for competitions or leisure. Prison-like conditions in single stables almost inevitably lead to psychological disturbances which, in certain cases, come to light years later.

As a herd animal that is instinctively poised for flight, the horse needs to be able to have some form of contact with other horses at all times for his emotional well-being. This need is fulfilled

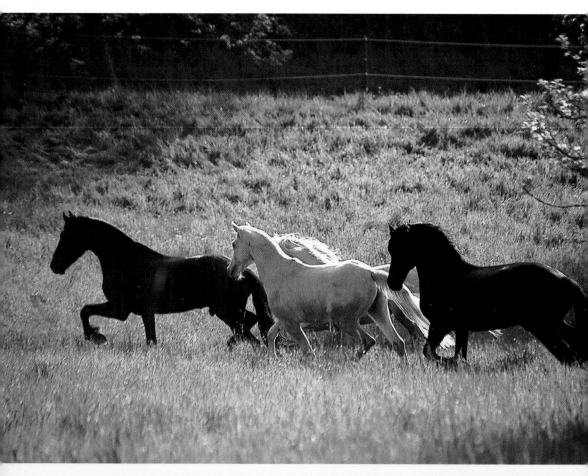

Every horse needs to be able to exercise daily with other horses for his psychological well-being. This is true of all horses whether they are competition horses or horses ridden for pleasure. Photo: Schmelzer

through actual physical contact with other horses, or by being able to see, hear, or smell them.

Being with the herd makes him feel secure and offers protection from enemies. For the horse, no man or other animal can replace his own kind.

There are several examples to prove the link between suitable stable management and the horse being used successfully at competitions. Psychologically balanced horses often display an outstanding ability to perform and are clearly less prone to illnesses. The responsibility lies with man, to modify his own beliefs so that his horse does not suffer any emotional or physical damage.

Suggestions for further reading and internet sites

Further reading

Bach Flower Remedies
Edward Bach
Keats Pub Inc

The Encyclopedia of Bach Flower Therapy
Mechthild Scheffer
Harper Collins

Inner Harmony Through Bach Flowers
Sigrid Schmidt
Time Life UK

Websites
www.nelsonspharmacy.com
www.bachfloweressences.co.uk

CADMOS
Equestrian

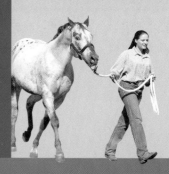

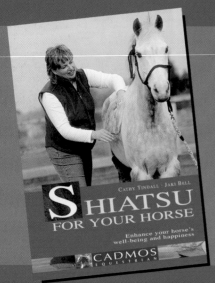

Cathy Tindall/Jaki Bell
SHIATSU FOR YOUR HORSE

In recent years the benefits of massage, physiotherapy and other 'touch' therapies to horses have become much better appreciated. Shiatsu is a traditional Japanese therapy based on pressure and stretches, the benefits of which you can share with your horse, enhancing his well-being and happiness.

This book is required reading for any horse owner or rider who want to give something back to these amazing, sensitive and understanding animals.

144 pages, hardback
ISBN 3-86127-915-0
£ 19,95

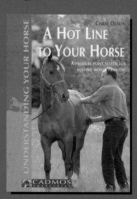

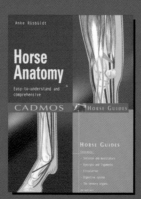

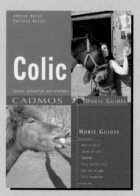

Chris Olson
A HOT LINE TO YOUR HORSE

Tension in horses is a common cause of loss performance, and impairs the harmonious cooperation of horse and rider. This book sets out an effective, easily comprehensible method which you can quickly master and use to enhance your horse's well-being and willingness to perform.

80 pages, paperback
ISBN 3-86127-901-0
£ 9,95

Anke Rüsbüldt
HORSE ANATOMY

Anyone who wants to care for and ride a horse well, needs to learn a few basics about anatomy. This guide explains the most important facts about anatomy in an easy and understandable way and helps the horse owner to communicate with their veterinary surgeon.

Anke Rüsbüldt is a practising veterinary surgeon specialising in equine medicine.

32 pages, paperback
ISBN 3-86127-951-7
£ 4,95

Andrea Holst/Daniela Bolze
COLIC

Colic is one of the main reasons for calling out the vet. It is a disease that must not be taken lightly, as it often proves fatal. This book explains the causes of colic, the symptoms of the various colic types – of which there are many – and particularly how to prevent colic. This is something every horse owner should know, because most colics can be prevented.

32 pages, paperback
ISBN 3-86127-945-2
£ 4,95

Cadmos Equestrian
171 GordonRoad   Nunhead
GB - London SE15 3RT
Tel.: 02074 504117   Fax: 08701 367219

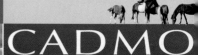

CADMO

CADMOS
Equestrian

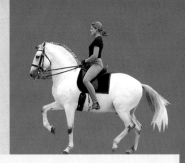

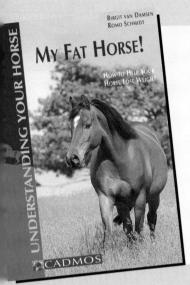

Birgit van Damsen/Romo Schmidt

MY FAT HORSE

Overweight horses are no rarity nowadays. Ponies and native breeds are often too heavy and are prone to weight related ailments. This book looks at the causes of obesity, and how to recognise it. It explains the dangers of obesity and offers solutions on how to reduce excess weight, examining diet, exercise and pasture management.
Birgit van Damsen is a journalist specialised in equine subjects and the author of several horse books.

80 pages, paperback
ISBN 3-86127-913-4
£ 9,95

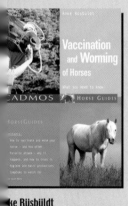

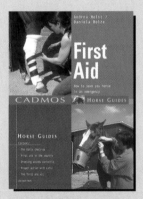

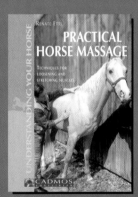

ke Rüsbüldt

ACCINATION AND ORMING OF HORSES

gular vaccination and worming pro-
ammes are of the utmost importance
your horse's health and general well-
ng. Looking at the mechanics of
ection and parasitic infestation, the
hor explains in detail why, how
en and against what you should
ccinate and worm.

ages, paperback
N 3-86127-931-2
95

Andrea Holst/Daniela Bolze

FIRST AID

Every rider should be prepared for an emergency. This guide describes how to treat the most frequent injuries and illnesses that occur, when to call the vet and what to do until the vet arrives. The authors describe how to bandage a wound in an emergency, what should be observed in the daily inspection for soundness, and much more.

32 pages, paperback
ISBN 3-86127-940-1
£ 4,95

Renate Ettl

PRACTICAL HORSE MASSAGE

This book provides a complete introduction to horse massage. It is a book for everyone who wants to help their horses to relax and regenerate after competitions or long rides. Renate Ettl is a horse therapist and trainer of Western riders. She lives in the south of Germany.

96 pages, paperback
ISBN 3-86127-903-7
£ 9,95

Cadmos Equestrian
171 GordonRoad   Nunhead
GB - London SE15 3RT
Tel.: 02074 504117   Fax: 08701 367219

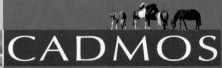
CADMOS

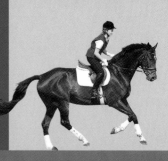
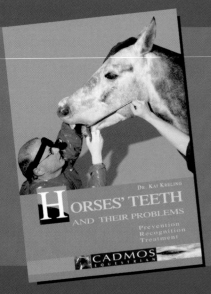
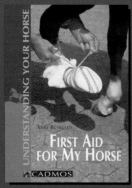
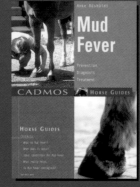
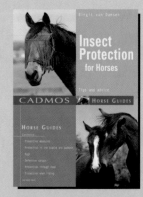

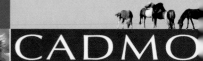